Better Than I Ever Expected

straight talk about sex after sixty

Joan Price

SEAL PRESS

Better Than I Ever Expected | Straight Talk about Sex after Sixty

Copyright © 2006 by Joan Price

For credits and additional copyright notices, see pages 268–269.

Some photos and illustrations are used by permission and are the property of the original copyright owners.

Published by
Seal Press
An Imprint of Avalon Publishing Group, Incorporated
1400 65th Street, Suite 250
AVALON
publishing group incorporated Emeryville, CA 94608

ISBN-10 1-58005-152-9
ISBN-13 978-1-58005-152-1

9 8 7 6 5 4 3 2 1

Library of Congress Cataloging-in-Publication Data
Price, Joan, 1943-
Better than I ever expected : straight talk about sex after sixty / Joan Price.
p. cm.
Includes bibliographical references.
ISBN-13: 978-1-58005-152-1 (pbk.)
ISBN-10: 1-58005-152-9 (pbk.)
1. Health. 2. Hormones. 3. Sex. 4. Vitality. I. Title.
RA776.5.P75 2006
613.9'54—dc22
2005023856

Cover and interior design by Amber Pirker
Printed in the United States of America by Malloy
Distributed by Publishers Group West

To my love, Robert Rice

Contents

Introduction

If I were asked for the major messages of this book, I'd shout out:

1. We are having hot, fabulous sex after sixty. Society's view of aging women as sexless is wrong, wrong, wrong. Many of us are having the best sex of our lives.

2. Yes, changes after menopause make sexual enjoyment challenging, but we're using our creativity, our personal power, the joy and intimacy of our relationships, and useful tools of all sorts—from sex toys to a sense of humor—to tackle those challenges.

3. We're redefining aging and sexuality. We're the Love Generation—we practically invented sex. We're not about to shut the gates now!

There are plenty of books and magazine articles filled with doom and gloom about midlife and older sexuality, how our tissues wither along with our libidos, and we might as well give it up. This isn't my book.

This book is more than a guide to how to have great sex after sixty—it's intensely personal, straight talk from my own experience and from a bevy of lusty women over sixty who aren't afraid to tell, along with a smattering of self-help tips from experts.

Most books about sex and older women are either academic or exclusively self-help. While we Boomers and beyond do want self-help, we are hungry for the voices of women's shared experiences. This book is warm, friendly, lighthearted, down-to-earth, often graphic, and honest.

I'm known as a fitness professional and health/fitness writer. I'm proud of the fitness books I've written, and just because I'm now writing about a new topic, it's not that I believe any less in the importance of exercise. (Notice how I sneak in a chapter on that theme in this book.)

But it's time—at age sixty-one—to expand my repertoire and dive into the subject that interests me the most at this stage of my life: ageless sexuality. Bodies beyond boundaries. From the reactions of the women I interviewed, we're eager to talk, and we're eager to learn from each other.

"I'm writing the book I'd love to read," I tell my friends. Now, in my sixties, I have the great joy of writing a book on my favorite topic of all time, and in the woman-to-woman-friendly style that I enjoy. May you join me in affirming and celebrating the joy in our sensual lives!

Joan Price
Sebastopol, California
2005

꙳ **CHAPTER 1**

Tale of a Book: How This Book Came to Be

History of This Book

In 2003, my book, *The Anytime, Anywhere Exercise Book: 300+ Quick and Easy Exercises You Can Do Whenever You Want!* came out. I was thrilled when my publicist phoned and said, "We may be able to book you on a TV program in New York called *Naked New York*. It's a cable show that discusses sex topics. Are any of your exercises especially good for sex?"

"Yes!" I replied.

"We need a hook, an angle," she said. "Something sexy about you."

"Tell them that at age fifty-nine, I'm having the best sex of my life!"

A month later, sitting in the studio waiting for my turn, I heard this promo before every commercial: "And coming up, Joan Price, who, at age fifty-nine, is having the best sex of her life!" I had thought this would be a minor attention-getter—I had no idea I'd sound like a freak.

During my fifteen minutes in the guest seat, I discovered that no one cared about my exercise book, though the host gave me about ten seconds to demonstrate exercises that strengthen the inner thighs and the woman-on-top push-up muscles. The major question of the evening was, "So, Joan, is it true that you're having the best sex of your life at fifty-nine? What makes it so good?"

My three-part answer was this:

1. We take lots and lots of time for sex—I need lots of warm-up, and we both enjoy it.

2. We know ourselves and our bodies, and we have learned how to communicate at this point in our lives.

3. My lover and I are in a new relationship. We're wildly in love with each other and feel like a couple of adolescents—but with the added eroticism that surprisingly accompanies wisdom and life experience.

How odd it felt to be disclosing intimate details of my sex life on television. Thank goodness my lover—an intensely private person—was safely across the country, where he couldn't hear me.

But, to tell the truth, I didn't mind talking about this at all. The fact was that I was in an amazing and intensely sexual relationship with Robert, age sixty-six at the time—who has since become my fiancé—and I was, indeed, having the best sex of my life. The glorious part is that it just keeps getting better! There's nothing hotter than sex between people who know their own bodies, are crazy about each other, relish taking lots of time, and honor sex as extremely spiritual and physical. I just don't think people can get there without a whole lot of life experience and a hefty dose of relationship mistakes along the way!

Me, Write a Sex Book?

When I was a young woman, it didn't occur to me that women over sixty cared about sex, much less tingled like teenagers in the presence of their lovers. The media do nothing to give us role models (see Chapter 2, "Sex in the Golden Age," for a discussion of this). We're staking out new territory here. Now that I had passed midlife, sex was different, to be sure, but wildly satisfying. Why didn't anyone tell me this would and could happen? Why weren't we talking about it? Why weren't we writing about it?

This idea kept percolating as I passed sixty, and I went looking for good sex books, both fiction and nonfiction, specifically aimed at my age group. I was surprised—and turned off!—by how few of these books existed, and how dry and unsexy most of them were. Some were much too academic to bring into the bedroom, many were outdated, and some were supposed to be titillating but weren't—at least to us.

I read the beginnings of several books to Robert in bed, trying to find one that would entice us, arouse us, or give us new insights, to no avail. "You should write your own book about sex and aging," Robert told me.

Yes, I thought. I could write a book that presents the reality of sex after sixty with all its challenges and delights. A book that celebrates sensuality, intimacy, and our marvelous bodies— sources of deep pleasures that transcend wrinkles and dryness. A book that isn't self-help as much as self-examination and self-revelation, though with a healthy sampling of strategies that help us make friends with our retreating hormones. A book that makes us laugh at ourselves. A book that makes us laugh just because we're happy!

> *We can still feel passionate about love, at any age, if the circumstances are right. Previous generations of older people would have gone into cardiac arrest if anyone had suggested such a thing; and most of us were probably brainwashed . . . to think we would become asexual zombies after sixty-five.*
> —Eda LeShan in *I Want More of Everything*[1]

Examine the Past, Understand the Present

I started writing memoir, a process I'd recommend to everyone. You don't have to aim to write a book—just start with a handwritten journal or a personal document on your computer and write down your thoughts and experiences.

As I did this, I gained in many ways: self-acceptance, new

perspectives on past relationships, insights about my values and attitudes, gratitude for the love in my life, and deep, reverent appreciation for this stage of my life.

As we skate our way along the path of life, we hit bumps, skid on unexpected curves, and push away brambles that obscure our vision. We're so intent on where we are and where we're headed that we don't always see clearly where we've been, or the impact a particular choice had on who we are now and how we feel about ourselves.

As I wrote this book, I found that remembering early experiences and people I had once invited into my life—and my bed—brought into vivid recall parts of my life that were truly formative. Loves budded, bloomed, and withered on the vine. I mourned, and I went on—to other loves, other blooms, and other endings.

That sounds pretty heavy. I also got in touch with the humor of my past experiences (even those I had mourned), my body, and my luscious relationship with my lover. I got to say whatever I wanted, however I wanted. I experienced great pleasure revisiting the good experiences and understanding the not-so-good choices in a new way. Often, when I returned to revise, I discovered a whole new way of looking at a particular part of my life, or the people who influenced me then.

Sisterhood Rediscovered

I knew it was important to present the voices of many women, not just my own. So I went in search of other women my age and older who were happy with their sexuality and had anecdotes, attitudes, and insights to share. I circulated this solicitation:

5

Sexually Seasoned Women Speak about What They Hope to Read in This Book

I want to know how other older women really feel about sex and what they do in private, and whether their experiences are similar to mine. I see a woman who looks my age or older, and I wish I could ask her, "So, what's your sex life like now?" *(Diana, 62)*

Many non-exotic tips and secrets I wouldn't have thought of myself that I would feel comfortable using. Dressing like a Playboy Bunny and similar tips wouldn't be right for me, but everyday ideas would be welcome. *(Tana, 60)*

Ideas for further enriching my sexual life. It would also be great to find out that fewer people are depriving themselves of the pleasures of sex because they think they're too old or that sex as an older person is somehow inappropriate. *(Mary Ann, 62)*

Wanted: Interviews with sassy, sexy women, age 60+, who are willing to share feelings and experiences openly and anonymously in a candid, woman-to-woman book.

My goodness, how willing they were to talk! I discovered that women sixty-plus are actively seeking the kind of community of other women—the sisterhood—that connected and supported us in the 1960s and 1970s. Women forwarded emails containing my interview requests to their friends and to mailing lists and message boards. The anonymity of cyberspace allowed a whole

Honesty about what keeps us going, the rewards of not giving up or giving in to changes in our bodies and our physical abilities, and that love and lovemaking are not just for the young. I would expect the hard truths about the reality of declining sexual appetites and abilities and the transition to a different kind of lovemaking perhaps, as well as some tools of the trade that come in handy to replace some of the lost abilities in each partner and stressing lovemaking over the "having intercourse" activities. *(Ulla, 61)*

Other women's stories popping out. Some bullet points that are fun, like "Ten of my favorite sex fantasies." *(Monica, 60)*

The truth, not a bunch of holier-than-thou bull. *(Catherine, 65)*

I'd like a lot of juicy stories and case histories. Forget the how-to. Make it frothy and entertaining. *(Erica, 62)*

new kind of networking. Women were hungry to talk about themselves and learn about each other.

The interviewing process was not designed to get any consensus of what sex is like for women after sixty, nor was it in any way a survey of experiences or attitudes. I'm no Kinsey researcher collecting data. Rather, I encouraged women to talk about topics relevant to their lives, in their own words.

Although some preferred to be interviewed by phone, most emailed their answers to me. They approached the questionnaire

with candor and enthusiasm, revealing intimate details of masturbation, affairs, and special sex rituals (with or without a partner),
entrusting me with their confidences with the click of the "send"
button. We often dialogued after that, as I requested more information or they thought of something else they wanted to share.
The process created a bond of woman-to-woman intimacy.

These wonderful women—most of them complete strangers
to me until the interview—were willing, even eager, to tell me
the most private details of their bodies, relationships, feelings,
and fantasies. Many shared experiences and thoughts that their
partners did not know. They expressed themselves creatively,
honestly—and sometimes juicily.

As intimately as these women spoke, I rarely heard profan-
ity or disrespectful terminology from these outspoken women
describing their private sex lives. They spoke and wrote with
dignity, a sense of reverence in their disclosures, respect for their
partners and themselves, a desire to communicate nuances by
choosing just the right word rather than the most expedient
street language.

In the late 1960s and early 1970s, we pondered our sexuality
and our relationships in communal gardens, coffee houses, and
consciousness-raising groups. Somehow we lost that connection
as we grew up—or maybe we just grew away. Now, more than
half a lifetime later, we are again sharing our thoughts, experiences, and feelings. It feels good.

What's in a Name?

The women who submitted interviews are identified in the
book by first names of their choice and their ages, and were

promised from the beginning that their identities would remain confidential, locked in my files. No one else has ever viewed their questionnaires, and not even my publisher knows who these women really are.

I am real, and everything I say about my experience is real. Robert is real. To protect their privacy, and often after consulting them, I have changed the names of most of the other people I mention in my own narrative, though not the details of the incidents.

On the Other Hand ...

I approached a woman in the gym, an outspoken, assertive woman I've known casually for years. She had always spoken openly about her boyfriends and once laughingly showed off her rug burn in the locker room after a vigorous encounter on the carpet. I told her about the book I was writing and asked if she'd like to be interviewed.

"Oh, I'm done with all that," she told me. "I'm so glad that's over. Now I have time to read a book."

"What if 80 percent of women *don't* feel enthusiastic about sex at our age?" a potential interviewee asked me. "Aren't you skewing the survey by only interviewing women who have a positive attitude about their sexuality?"

This isn't a survey, I explained, and sure, there are women (I don't claim to know what percent) who are happy to be done with sex, like my gym acquaintance. Yes, several people told me they were not having good sex when I asked if they wanted to be interviewed, and certainly many more took themselves out of the running because of the wording I used to solicit interviews. Several women told me their intimate lives were too private to

---

Sexually Seasoned Women Speak about Being Interviewed about Their Sex Lives

I love talking about this stuff. It's my favorite topic. *(Erica, 62)*

I was surprised to find how strongly my joy in life is connected to the joy in my sexual life. It also reinforced my appreciation for the remarkable man I married. *(Mary Ann, 62)*

It was fun to answer this. I just worry that someone might recognize me. Gulp! *(Melanie, 64)*

Fun! Fun! Fun! It's so nice to talk about these things with someone who actually wants to hear about it. My friends think I'm crazy or obsessed *(or both)*, and my kids just plain don't want to hear about it. Especially when I mention younger men. *(Kaycee, 66)*

---

reveal in a book, even anonymously—but they wanted to read the book when it came out.

Writing about It, Doing It, Writing about Doing It

"Isn't this better than writing about sex?" Robert whispers into my hair as we snuggle after a sunny, stolen afternoon of magnificent lovemaking.

Yes, of course, doing it is better than writing about sex! But in my mind, I'm writing about it all the time, inviting sensations

Being anonymous made it easy to be completely honest. (My friends know how I think and what I believe, but I figure there's no sense telling the whole world.) *(Catherine, 65)*

It feels nice to talk about my sex life—and it's been a little bit of a soul-searching experiment in sticking to being honest. *(Ulla, 61)*

It's kind of a turn-on to be writing about my sex life. I'm a bit embarrassed for my husband to read what I wrote, but I'll probably let him. *(Penny, 60)*

What a surprise—someone wants me to talk about sex after sixty. I would be more than happy to tell the world about such joy. I can be open with you because you understand, or you wouldn't be writing this book to hopefully wake up some folks. Thanks for being a writer in our world. *(Claire, 66)*

and forming words that I might use to describe the experience. Knowing that my computer waits for my words is a turn-on, not a distraction, an intensification of sensation because I'm so completely focused on it.

And the act of writing about sex is erotic. I replay sensual details through my mind and decide which ones to offer publicly. As I pluck the right words to depict a sexy thought or memory, I often find myself wriggling in my ergonomic chair, anticipating the next time I close down the computer and turn my attention to my lover. It is titillating to translate sexual experiences into words, capturing snippets of conversation, whiffs of sensual detail, metaphors of touch, and verses of the songs of love.

Robert: Where Did My Privacy Go?

"Do you really have to write about that?" Robert asks me, squirming at the details I've revealed in a chapter I'm reading to him. "You know I'm really a private person."

He imagines his son and daughter, the line dancers we teach, and his artist friends reading about the secret message of his nail-filing and other exchanges of sensual love that he never thought would be revealed beyond the immediacy of our two bodies. He jokingly contemplates disguises he'll wear after the book comes out. But I know this playfulness cloaks a serious concern.

"It's only because I love you and respect your work that I'm taking on this challenge of seeing so much of our intimacy broadcast to the public," Robert says in one of our many talks about what to reveal and what to leave under the covers. I read each chapter to him before I submit it to my editor. Sometimes I ask his permission to include a detail I'd like to disclose. He knows I treat our private life with reverence as much as candor. He also knows when I strip the covers off the bed and show what's going on frankly, I do it respectfully.

"Honestly, I'm not fully comfortable with you revealing so much, but I know how important this book is to you, and to your readers," Robert continues. "As an abstract artist, I know the courage it takes to forge a new direction that may not be supported, even by friends and colleagues. You sometimes say things with a directness of language that surprises me, that's less refined than I might want to use. But I don't want to restrict what you feel needs to be said. At this time in my life, I feel as prepared as I'll ever be to handle this kind of challenge. Ultimately, it's the act of honoring truth and an opportunity for me to continue to grow. Besides, what you're doing is important."

Between the Covers

I continue to devour other writers' books about sex in general and sex after menopause in particular. I don't find much about sex after sixty. I want to be able to recommend other books to you if they're especially good, and of course I want to know what else is out there.

Not long ago, I was notified that fifteen books I had requested from my local library had arrived. Realize that Sebastopol, California, is a smallish town, and I've been frequenting the local library for thirty years. Most of the librarians know me by name. I felt I owed the fifty-something librarian an explanation when I hoisted fifteen books with "sex" in the title onto the checkout counter. "I'm writing a book called *Better Than I Ever Expected: Straight Talk about Sex after Sixty*," I explained.

"Good!" she exclaimed. "I knew by the time I got there, the book I needed would be waiting for me!"

Redefining This Aging Stuff: Are We on TV Yet?

I take a break from writing and channel surf. Three different television talk shows feature the sexiness of older women! One teaches women to pole dance and strip for their husbands. Another performs a clothing makeover, trading in sweats for La Perla lingerie. A third presents a discussion of a book featuring "cougars": older

Sexually Seasoned Women Speak about What They Wish Other Women Understood about Sex after Sixty

Sex after sixty is not only okay, it is critical to your balanced well-being. Sex is something you are, not just something you do. *(Kendall, 69)*

I wish women knew to keep loving their own bodies, to keep expecting to be treated like a sexy, beautiful woman. What we expect, we get. *(Monica, 60)*

Don't let this life pleasure get away from you—work at it. It's worth it! Keep your partner primary in your life. Stay in touch with his sexual interests as well as your own, let him know what you like and how you like it done, and listen to him as he does the same. *(Mary Ann, 62)*

It's a matter of getting ourselves to a place where we think we deserve to be sexually happy. Getting that self-esteem thing going and having it apply to sex as well as to everything else in our life. When people bloom, their sex lives stay good. *(Nina, 67)*

Looks and age are not so important. Who we are is vital. I look at my birth certificate, and I'm a realist. I won't pretend to be what I'm not in order to have a man in my life. But if the Goddess should be so kind as to put one in my pathway, then I will enjoy him and celebrate him and worship God in him as best I can. If you've got a reasonably attentive partner, rejoice and give thanks. If not, rejoice in the simplicity of your life. *(Rachel, 62)*

Younger men are turned on by us. Experience and a free-spirited attitude are very important. *(Phoebe, 64)*

What joy a good and kind sexual partner brings into our lives. At this age, we all need to own those desires, be grateful for them, and be so happy that our bodies are healthy enough to want to have sex. Zelda Fitzgerald once said that "looking for love is like asking for a new point of departure in life," and looking for sexual pleasure is a good thing to take on that journey. *(Claire, 66)*

Keep an open mind. Remember that there is always something new to try and so many men out there. Sex after sixty could be the best time of your life if you play it right. *(Kaycee, 66)*

The second part of our lives begins at sixty, and it is better than the first part. *(Lily, 60)*

After sixty, it's not downhill. It's still uphill when it comes to sex, only just like a car, it slows down just a little and the hill may seem a little steeper sometimes. *(Ulla, 61)*

Too darn much emphasis is put on age when it's only a number. You are still a hot woman, and you don't need a man to validate you. If you're feeling horny, think sexy thoughts and stimulate yourself. If you see someone you want, go for it, but please use safe sex. *(Catherine, 65)*

women in relationships with younger men. You'd think that our society is finally ready for us sassy older women!

Listen and look carefully, though, and you see that the "older" women teaching these lessons to the rest of us are probably in their forties max! "You ain't seen nothing yet!" I yell at the midlife women who think they're experts on sex and aging.

Of course, it's hard to tell how old these women really are, with their lean, hard bodies, tight facial skin, and absence of wrinkles, all of which reveal little about age these days, thanks to exercise, cosmetics, and the prevalence of "procedures." After all, many of us sixty-something women have legs as youthful looking as the ones on this book cover, thanks to step aerobics, hiking, and dancing.

Still, I'd like to see women who admit that (and look like) they're over sixty on these talk shows, rousing other older women to assert their sexuality—as the women I interviewed have done. Perhaps we'll do that together.

I enjoy the thought that little by little, we'll accept that women can and do stay sexy through the decades, and it doesn't stop when we can no longer hide the wrinkles or saggy skin.

I make this prediction: By the time this book has been out a year, there will be so many additional books, magazine articles, and talk shows on this theme that we'll barely remember when we were expected to retreat into asexuality.

≈ **CHAPTER 2**

Sex in the Golden Age

Age is something that doesn't matter, unless you are a cheese.
—Billie Burke

Sexuality Is Not Age-Bound

What makes sex after sixty the best sex of our lives? Our bodies might be aging, but great sex isn't just about body parts. When we've got wisdom, connection, logistics, time, intimacy, a sense of humor, ease of communication, resilience of body and spirit, and no kids barging in, who needs youth?

Sexual response is in our brains more than our genitals. We

can have the best sex of our lives at our age, largely because we know ourselves deeply by now. We know who we are and what we want both in and out of bed. We've made—and continue to make—significant life choices. We understand intimacy and what we want in a sex partner and a life partner. We choose partners who are more mature, wiser, and interested in a deeper, more spiritual connection—interested in us as complex human beings. We've learned to communicate.

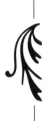 *Life's under no obligation to give us what we expect.*
—Margaret Mitchell

Life's Surprises

When I discovered sex at seventeen with my first love, I had firm beliefs about what sex, love, and life would offer me. I would never have believed any guardian angel or gypsy fortune-teller who told me, "Right now, you love your young man with your whole being, but you will love others as much, differently each time, changing and growing with each new relationship and each period of solitude. Finally, you will meet your ultimate love when you're fifty-seven and continue having the best sex of your life after sixty."

I not only would have rejected this prediction out of disbelief, I would have shuddered at the idea of a sixty-year-old having sex! And who'd want to read about it, even if I were crazy enough to do it and admit to it?

Now, decades later, I discover that I am, at sixty-one, an intensely sexual being, capable of the most powerful physical and spiritual love that I have ever experienced. And I find a huge community of women who want to share their experiences and learn about each other's.

What Do We Want at This Stage of Our Lives?

Many of us have lived our lives as self-propelled, go-getter women with full, fast-paced, goal-driven lives revolving around work, family, money, relationships, and a million concerns and duties. Around menopause, many of us took a hard look at how we wanted to be spending our energy. Many of us made both big and little changes to steady our roller-coaster lives.

One friend made a gym locker room of women laugh when she announced, "Menopausal memory is actually a relief—I don't have to be the memory repository for my whole family! I just told my husband and teenage kids, 'Remember your own darn appointments and obligations—I'm not doing it for you anymore.'"

After months of menopausal sleep deprivation, I told the health club where I taught group exercise that I was no longer willing to teach the 6:00 AM step class. Although I used to wake up when it was light and go to sleep when it got dark, just like a chicken, menopause turned me into a night owl, and switching my teaching and exercising scheduling from morning aerobics to evening line dancing intensified that change. A whole new world opened up socially when I saw 9:00 PM as midevening instead of the middle of the night.

Now, with the menopause years or decades behind us, we

Sexually Seasoned Women Speak about What They—as Young Women—Expected from Sex after Sixty

I figured it'd all be over, that I'd be sitting on the porch crocheting doilies or doing good works. I'd probably have thought it would be disgusting to engage in sex with an aging body. Back then, it was all about looking good and being desirable. *(Rachel, 62)*

Sex got better and better as time passed, and it really didn't occur to me that it might go away. At the same time, I certainly doubted my parents or in-laws had an active sex life! *(Mary Ann, 62)*

I didn't know that older women could even have sex, let alone climax. I remember my ex-husband's mother at sixty-five telling me that she and her husband had no sex after sixty. I thought, *Oh, what a dirty old woman for being interested at her age! (Bea, 77)*

continue to strive to get in touch with what makes for a balanced life. Many of us are still goal-driven, but our goals may be different—more about personal connections than bank balances. We see our own mortality, and that impels us to examine exactly what we need in our lives to be fulfilled at this stage and where we need to take time to nurture ourselves. Personally and professionally, I've stopped doing things I don't want to do—life's too short, too full, and

I never expected that it would get worse. I'm having sex, and I'm enjoying it. The stuff that's out there in society is very sex-negative for older people. *(Nina, 67)*

I guess I thought I would always want sex, but didn't think anyone would want me. *(Joanna, 61)*

I wondered if I'd have any. When I was with my husband and I had a headache, he'd tell me, "Someday you'll be sorry." *(Matilda, 78)*

I thought our frequency would drop off precipitously, but it's been only a slight decrease, despite the fact that neither of us is as "responsive" as we were decades ago. *(Tana, 60)*

I never thought that sex at my age would be so important. I had what I thought was a game plan for this stage of my life, and now sex is number one. And I love it! *(Kaycee, 66)*

too important to waste—and I make time for the important activities and the people I love.

For many of us, that translates to a good, hot, loving, self-indulgent, sexual relationship.

Even that word "self-indulgent" tries to make me feel guilty, but I don't let it. If I can't take time for myself now, when can I? If I don't shove aside work to spend an exuberant afternoon with my virile and tender lover, when will I? What's more important than nurturing the hottest, sweetest, and most fulfilling relationship that I've ever had?

According to the Research

Research on older women and sexuality was sparse until recently, but it is now kicking into high gear as Boomers (and their doctors and therapists) look for clues. As we await their conclusions, let's peek at two older studies that validate our experiences and tell us much about ourselves and, in some cases, our culture:

• 70 percent of sexually active women over sixty reported being as satisfied or more satisfied with their sexual lives than they were in their forties, according to a 1998 survey of nearly 1,300 Americans aged sixty or older, conducted by the National Council on the Aging.[1] My experience certainly supports that. In my forties, I was unnerved by the realization that my sex life was being affected by undeniable signs and feelings of aging. Now I've grown past wanting to hold onto youth in the bedroom, and as a result I feel truly present with my lover and capable of intense satisfaction.

• 84 percent of older females in 106 cultures studied in 1982 exhibited continued sexual activity and expressions of strong sexual interest. "The continuance of sexuality in many societies during aging and the limitation of sexuality in other societies suggests that cultural as well as biological factors may be key determinants in sexual behavior in the later part of life."[2] How refreshing to get this validation that the sexless crone image is a product of our culture's anti-age bias, not our biology or destiny.

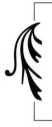

> *The Baby Boomer generation has never been*
> *known for passively accepting models for living*
> *handed down from prior generations.*
>
> —Sheryl A. Kingsberg, PhD[3]

Thank You, Dr. Kingsberg

We all know that aging brings about hormonal and other physical changes in women, some of which send our sex drive careening downward. So how can we claim to be having great sex during a time of lowered sex drive? What is propelling our intense sexual interest and satisfaction at the same time that our physical arousal seems more elusive?

"Drive" is only one component of "desire," points out researcher Sheryl A. Kingsberg, PhD, in her 2000 study, "The Impact of Aging on Sexual Function in Women and Their Partners." Stay with me here, this is important: Kingsberg explains that "drive" is the biologic impetus to have sex, and that's the part that's likely flagging in our aging bodies. However, "desire" is drive plus two additional, extremely important components:

1. beliefs/values about sex, which influence how much we want to behave sexually, and

2. psychological/interpersonal motivation, which influences how much we want to be sexual with a certain partner.

This hit me with an "Aha!" when I read Kingsberg's study. So, I'm having the most wonderfully satisfying sex despite slowing physiological responses because (in my own words now):

• I love and desire my partner: the whole person he is, his gorgeous body, and the physical and emotional parts of our intimacy.

Sexually Seasoned Women Speak about Pulling the Mattress into the Empty Nest

Yahoo! Freedom to bring home anyone I wanted, and he could stay the night. I could go away for weekends with no one to answer to or worry about. *(Catherine, 65)*

When I was younger with kids in the house, I remember always trying not to make too much noise. But now? Making a lot of noise adds to the pleasure—quite a bit! *(Aurora, 60)*

We no longer had to be as careful in case one of the kids would come in. That happened once in the afternoon, so embarrassing! My husband and I had been to a wedding and had champagne. We were in the bedroom, and we didn't lock the door. My twelve-year-old son walked in on my husband giving me oral sex. He opened the door and turned around and walked out. We never talked about it. *(Jaime, 73)*

We had another honeymoon. We were like kids again. We lived in New York and played tourist. It was a very nice time. We had a life. We had time to travel and do things. *(Matilda, 78)*

• I'm happy with myself and my own life independent of this relationship.

• I enjoy my body, its strength and sensations, and its ability to move and respond.

The additional privacy gave us considerably more freedom to talk openly, tease each other, and play. It also extended the time we set aside for a glass of wine and dinner before we'd shower and head for bed. *(Mary Ann, 62)*

Greater privacy meant greater spontaneity. *(Tana, 60)*

Since we both work at home, it suddenly became possible to have sex in the morning (instead of having to jump out of bed and take care of the kids' needs) and at any other time of day. *(Pepper, 71)*

My four children are spread out over fifteen years, so it is only recently that I had an empty nest. My husband and I both enjoy the privacy and the ability to be spontaneous about sex. We have had a few funny and annoying episodes when kids dropped in unexpectedly. *(Susie, 60)*

When the kids left, it really gave me a whole new sense of freedom and adventure. I don't really enjoy having sex when there are other people in the house. *(Penny, 60)*

I felt freer about having sex in various parts of the house and enjoyed being nude around the house. *(Ulla, 61)*

Honey, the Kids Are Gone!

On a more mundane plane, the logistics of sex are far easier for most of us. We have more leisure time to explore long, languid afternoon delights. There's no fear of pregnancy or of kids barging in. We don't need to serve dinner at dinnertime if we feel like making love through the evening. I never had children, so I'll invite the women I interviewed to describe the pleasures of sex after the kids move out in the sidebar on the previous pages.

> *If you use the media as your sole indicator . . . all the longhaired lover boys and mini-skirted chicks of the 1960s . . . lost their prodigious former libido [when they hit sixty]. The orgasm must surely, a flick through any newspaper or magazine will show, be exclusively the privilege of young, firm-fleshed people.*
>
> —Jonathan Margolis in
> *O: The Intimate History of the Orgasm*[4]

Boo Hiss Department

We're bombarded with media messages that older sex is unseemly, embarrassing, pathetic, ludicrous, and altogether icky. If television and movies allude to older people having sex at all (which they usually don't), the audience is invited to shudder, laugh, or bolt. We seldom see older people celebrating their sexuality. *Something's Gotta Give* is a stellar exception.

I used to try to ignore this attitude, but now I'm taking a more defiant stand. I've started a collection of examples so that we can rally together to boo and hiss and feel better. Please send your nominees for the "Boo Hiss Department," as well as examples of acceptance of older age sexuality (they're coming, I know they are), to joan@joanprice.com for a future edition.

• In an episode of *House,* a television medical drama that I usually like, we were supposed to laugh and recoil when a pelvic exam revealed that an older woman was having more consensual sex than her aged vagina could handle. Then—shock of shocks—we discovered that the Viagra-enhanced couple was having an extramarital affair! I guess we were supposed to laugh some more when Dr. House verbally humiliated them. I didn't.

• A young male comedian on television joked that older men needed Viagra, not because they were unable to perform but because older women were so ugly. Women in the audience laughed as much as the men.

• A *Denver Post* columnist was grateful that the bared-belly fashion fad seemed to be passing and noted that no woman over forty should have worn that style to begin with, no matter how good she looked. Oh? Is it better to see prepubescent girls sexualizing themselves with bare navels than women over forty who presumably are secure enough in their sexuality and their workout-sculpted abs to decide whether to show them off? (No, I don't bare my own midriff—it's the principle of the thing that I'm arguing.)

• On *Ally McBeal,* a hit television show of the 1990s, a young male lawyer had a fetish for older women's "wattles" (the extra skin on their necks), especially those of a sixty-ish judge, Dyan Cannon. Cannon is a beautiful woman, but we were directed to focus on her sagging skin.

• On *The Practice,* another sixty-ish judge, Holland Taylor, was portrayed as a post-menopausal nymphomaniac who seduced younger lawyers.

• In *Searching for Debra Winger,* a documentary by Rosanna Arquette, Winger and other film actresses discussed age discrimination against women in their profession, professing that men "as ugly as Mr. Potato Head" with "a face like a foot" can get serious acting roles where they can do great work, "but there are no regular-looking women."

• Doris Roberts, three-time Emmy winner for her role in the CBS comedy *Everybody Loves Raymond*, told the Associated Press in 2005 that she didn't know what she'd be doing after the end of the show's nine-year run because "Nobody writes for older people."

• On Jerry Hall's "reality" show *Kept*, men in their twenties compete for the honor of becoming the boy-toy escort of Hall, age forty-eight. They give the supermodel, actress, and ex of Mick Jagger personalized gifts, swim in a cold river, write poems, tell her lies, behave well at dinner parties, and variously vie for her affections, a moment of fame, and a hefty salary. Is this the only way an older woman can get a date, even a procedure-enhanced former supermodel? Give me a break!

The media give us few positive role models. I was delighted by the script and Diane Keaton's performance in *Something's Gotta Give*, but why was the theme of this movie such a rarity? Why do most midlife actresses have to either reinvent themselves through plastic surgery or resign themselves to roles as sexless crones? As Goldie Hawn's character in *The First Wives Club* said, "There are only three ages of women in Hollywood: babe, district attorney, and *Driving Miss Daisy*."

Maybe, just maybe, as Boomers slide into their redefinition of older-age sexuality, our culture's attitudes will change. We've made a difference in just about every other societal stereotype we've butted up against so far; why stop now?

Recently, I videotaped Sophia Loren in a Larry King interview for Robert, knowing he finds her one of the sexiest women ever.

"Whoa," he kept saying, voice deep, eyes glued to her beautifully aged face and cleavage. Even her eyeglasses were sexy. (Of course, if you looked like Sophia Loren when you were thirty, your chances of looking like a bombshell in your sixties are pretty good.)

More Media Musings

On the eve of my thirtieth birthday, I watched *The Graduate*, in which Anne Bancroft seduced Dustin Hoffman, who was dating her own daughter. I remember thinking my youth was over because I identified with Mrs. Robinson and experienced a great surge of compassion for her attraction to younger men. And as sexy as her legs were, we were supposed to see her as a pathetic example of an older woman gone emotionally astray and sexually over the top.

I discover now that Bancroft was only thirty-five and Hoffman was thirty when they made this film in 1966.

I think back about other film portrayals of sexual older women:

• *Harold and Maude* (1971): The odd-couple relationship between youthful Harold and eighty-year-old Maude is touching and original, but are we supposed to see Maude as a frisky elder living life as passionately as possible or a cartoon-character, old-lady kook? If the former, why did she have to kill herself at the peak of her zest?

• *Cocoon* (1985): Old folks discover a rejuvenating swimming pool and suddenly get frisky, break-dancing and having sex all over the place. They overuse the pool, the waters lose their powers, and the old folks are back where they started, except some are divorced or dead. A morality lesson?

• Mae West (1893–1980) was in a class by herself. She played sexpots in movies when she was in her forties and continued playing the curvy, sassy, lusty, and lusted-after woman in films and plays into her eighties, always surrounded by young male admirers. Although toward the end she became a caricature of herself, she embodied the power, zest, and humor of female libido.

BOO HISS PRIZE

Erica, Sixty-two, Sounds Off about Hollywood's Portrayals of Older Women:

Let's give a Boo Hiss prize to Hollywood in general for featuring older men as sexual beings and not giving parts to older women at all, unless it's as a mom or grandmom. The older men are almost always romancing women at least twenty years younger without the age disparity ever being mentioned. Believe it, if there were a movie with a sixty-year-old woman romantically involved with a forty-year-old man, it would be a very different story.

There is still rampant prejudice against older-age sexuality, mostly directed toward women, and it's so much a part of our culture that it's not even noticed. That's why the Diane Keaton film was such a phenomenon, because it was so rare to see a woman her age being sexual. In Hollywood as a rule, older male actors are still considered sexy while women are all discarded in their forties. Think Jack Nicholson, Paul Newman, Clint Eastwood, Harrison Ford—even Woody Allen has the chutzpah to cast himself as a the lover of women thirty years his junior.

It is only when you are at childbearing age that physical appearance is important. Once you are beyond procreation, you relate more as human beings. The male/female pairing off goes on, but it is more spiritual—less to do with lust and more to do with love, which is not a bad thing.

—Fay Weldon

Spirituality of Older Sex

As we get older and more in touch with reflection and spiritual self-examination, we affirm (or perhaps discover for the first time) the spirituality of sex. We are affirming:

1. our bodies, the exaltation of touch, sensation, the ability to feel pleasure,

2. our connection with our partner, which goes far beyond the physical, and

3. our resilience, because despite physical and emotional aches

I can now use sex as a spiritual and self-awareness practice. It was harder to find sophisticated partners who knew how to reach a high level of arousal, a practice of Tantra, when I was younger. I did know two men like this in my twenties and thirties—but they were older men. —Bess, 63

Sexually Seasoned Women Speak about Why Golden-Age Sex Is "Better Than I Ever Expected"

I have an incredible partner. He's so loving and has been such an amazing partner in my life. He's twelve years younger than I am, and I met him at forty-two. I was in peri-menopause, and our sex was the hottest you can imagine. We didn't get out of bed for days. We got married when I was forty-five, and I went into the deep, dark stuff of menopause. He's a poet and loves the feminine. Everything about our life and our sex life is about the feminine being honored. *(Monica, 60)*

The best thing about sex now is being relaxed and open with my partner. He has been with enough women that I know anything I do would not shock him. As a young woman, I was reluctant to tell a man what I liked. Now, at this age, I find these older men are very adept at finding out your secret wishes. The more my boyfriend pleases me, the more eager I am to reciprocate. It's too bad some men haven't figured this out. *(Melanie, 64)*

It's definitely a two-way street, giving and taking. Women have the greatest capacity for nurturing, and giving freely to our partners may take a little energy, but the payback is multifold. Keeping sex stimulating and satisfying empowers women in the relationship in amazing ways and makes everything so much more fun. Being flirtatious and sexy, even at the most subtle level, makes us feel better and younger. All that experience of years of sex shouldn't go to waste: Now it's a piece of cake—we know what it takes. What could be better than to have your partner keep falling in love with you more and more? *(Ulla, 61)*

The best thing about sex at my age is the ability to release inhibitions. I am increasingly accepting of the fact that sex is natural and can be talked about. This year I shocked a friend and one of our sons by alluding to our sex life openly. *(Pepper, 71)*

Maturity has a lot to do with it. I know more what to expect and what I expect. When you're coming up through the ranks, there are a lot of unexpected moments. That's still nice, but to know what to expect is very satisfying. To know that you can receive what you can expect. That you can count on your partner to know what you want. *(Leona, 77)*

I am overwhelmed and amazed that at sixty-six, I will probably have more fun having sex than ever before. I have always been a sexual person. Being a sensual/sexual person on this planet is my right and something I will never feel shame about again. I've just now met this woman who is in the same place—we are willing to share with each other everything we've known and everything else that we want to try. There's a feeling of excitement, and there's no hiding. *(Claire, 66)*

I have a lover thirty years younger. *(Bea, 77)*

and pains, we are—yes!—still capable of climbing the heights of sex and love.

For me, at this age, the real special secret to great sex is love. I've gone from a firm believer in impetuous sex in my youth to mature love, love that's only possible after a lot of life experience and probably a lot of wrong relationships along the way. Robert is the man I've been waiting for my whole life, and it's my enormous joy to have the pleasure of loving him and being loved by him. Sex blossoms rather than explodes these days.

CHAPTER 3

My Sex Education

I married the first man I ever kissed. When I tell my children that, they just about throw up.

—Barbara Bush

Birds and Bees, Pistils and Stamens

I was twelve, with budding breasts, when my father—an obstetrician/gynecologist—sat me down and handed me a pamphlet about the "facts of life." It was 1955, and the language was vague, with references to pistils and stamens and very little about penises or vaginas. There was certainly no reference to the clitoris. The only fully developed information was about how the egg in the woman was fertilized by the sperm from the man, leading to pregnancy. My father sat quietly as I, embarrassed and confused, read the pamphlet.

"Do you have any questions?" he asked when I finished.

"No," I lied.

I did have one burning question, which I asked my best friend: "How does the sperm get from the man to the woman?" That itty-bitty fact was nowhere in the pamphlet.

My friend, oh so much wiser, told me, "He puts *it* in her."

Whoa. I could barely believe it. All those pregnant women in my father's office—they had let their husbands put *it* in them? My own parents had done this? At least *twice?* (I had one brother.) I myself would have to permit this if I wanted to have children after I was married?

Not only was "how" omitted from my introduction to sexual information, but also "why." Over the next few years, I was taught what not to do (sex or anything that could lead to it) and what awful things could happen—after all, my father saw lives ruined by teenage pregnancy. I was never taught why people *want* to have sex and how fulfilling it can be.

I was totally unprepared for the excitement and delicious pleasure of my urges a few years later.

First Love

I fell in love with Donny in 1958, at fifteen. I was a shy, short kid—under five feet tall—and a sophomore in high school. He was a dashing, handsome, popular senior, six feet tall, with deep, dark eyes that stirred parts of me I hadn't known existed. We dated, laughed, shared confidences, held hands, and kissed and petted through the next two years. We were crazy in love. Just seeing him made my virgin heart and other organs throb.

We planned to marry after college, and we both intended to remain virgins until then, as our upbringing had instilled in us. But the hormones beckoned, and, after all, we were in love. At age seventeen, I left virginity behind. For the next year and a half, we were lovers.

But despite our enthusiasm and our love, I never had an orgasm. We didn't know how! We thought if our intercourse was harder, or slower, or gentler, or faster, it would happen.

I looked for information in books, but the books we needed—if they existed at all at that time—weren't in libraries. The few sex books I found didn't show the clitoris. I didn't even know I had one, much less what to do with it. I was so naive that I didn't know that girls could masturbate, so I never discovered my sweet spot myself.

I just knew that intercourse, however extended, in this position or that, got me high and was intensely pleasurable but never took me over the top. I didn't feel frustrated—I didn't really know what was missing (the ghastly name at the time for women like me was "frigid"). I loved sex, thought about it all the time, and wanted to do it whenever we had the chance. I still think lovingly about Donny and am grateful for being introduced to sex in such a caring way. Orgasm just was never a part of it.

Frequency also was never a part of it because we had to sneak and hide, and we rarely had unsupervised solitude or access to a bed. We made good use of the couch in a local business where I worked part-time during high school and had a key. It is amazing to me now that we got away with our after-hours shenanigans and that no other employee ever returned to work at night (or to pursue his or her own extracurricular activities!) to find us there.

Getting Caught

The summer after I graduated from high school, my parents— not trusting me not to do what they didn't know I was already doing—sent me off to a resort in the Catskills with my grandmother. Oh, the dullness of an old-people's resort (as I saw it then) for an eighteen-year-old separated from her boyfriend! I promptly got sick and stayed sick all summer, pining for Donny and writing letters to him from my sickbed, describing exactly what activities and body parts I was yearning for.

My grandmother took advantage of having a feverish, captive audience by sitting at my bedside, lecturing me about virginity. "If you let a man have his way with you before marriage, he'll never marry you!" she told me, wagging her finger in my face. "After all, why buy the cow when you get the milk free?" My mother, she told me, had been a "virgin through and through" until her marriage to my father. I pondered the "through and through" part.

To make a long story a little shorter, my grandmother snagged one of my letters to Donny before it hit the outgoing mail and learned in no uncertain terms that her lecture had been too late. She pocketed the letter to save for my parents. I knew nothing about this.

That fall, I went off to Bennington College, and one day I was surprised by a visit from my father. "I've read your letter to Donny," he told me as we sat in his car. I felt our loving, sweet, *private* relationship was being dragged through the mud, soiled and judged by people who had no right to view it.

"Who was the aggressor?" he asked—the oddest question I could imagine. I asked him to return my letter. "It was pornographic," he replied. "I burned it."

He told me that the two of us were never to see each other except when supervised by either my parents or his. Of course we ignored this and learned to sneak even more efficiently, but this invasion scared and scarred us both.

Donny Looks Back

I phoned Donny—with whom I have stayed in touch over the decades—to tell him about this book and what I wanted to write about him. We reminisced about our romance and the importance of it to us both. "I don't know if I ever told you this," Donny confided. "Your father called me for a private meeting and said he could have me put in jail. He told me I needed to straighten out, think about what I was doing." No, I hadn't known that.

I invited Donny to write his reminiscences about our relationship and our sexual explorations. He wrote this:

> To me, our relationship was a revelation and something I still cherish. I remember your concern about satisfaction, and I remember my concern about your concern. Was I doing something wrong? As a male, orgasm was just a natural part of the deal—not something I had to work at to achieve. But I remember feeling an obligation to you to make the experience as satisfying as I could. Of course, since we were learning by doing, I didn't know what I should be

doing to please you. And I really wanted to. I guess this led to some underlying frustration.

As far as knowing anything about the opposite sex, I was totally in the dark, as were my friends. We just had a lot of curiosity but no knowledge. We talked among ourselves, as I'm sure you did with your friends—although girls were more into sharing than we boys were.

I never got any input from my parents or family, nothing from school (it was the fifties), nothing I remember from books. So—I learned by doing. Exciting, confusing, dangerous.

From my point of view, I was making love to the most fantastic girl/woman in the whole world. You were an oasis. Making love to you was the sweetest part of a very satisfying relationship in all respects—except that we had to sneak around and be very cautious about what we did and where we did it.

Forty Years Later

My father's and grandmother's actions were clearly wrong and caused me much pain. But I finally realize that holding onto that pain after forty years says more about me than about them. They were victims of their own upbringing, and they thought they were doing the right thing—protecting me, loving me in the way they knew how.

I finally see that it's time for me to forgive and move on. I feel compassion for my parents and grandmother for not having escaped from the confines of their narrow views about sexuality, and I can imagine how stifling and unfulfilling this must have

Sexually Seasoned Women Speak about Early Sex Ed and Experiences

I was reared in a home where one did not talk about sex. When I first had sex at nineteen, I felt guilty because I was raised to believe it was something for married people. However, my guilt did not stop me. I justified it by becoming engaged. *(Melanie, 64)*

It seems like those who taught us about sex forget to tell us just how pleasurable it is. *(Kaycee, 66)*

We need to remember how the fear of pregnancy kept us from enjoying sex when we were younger. In the 1950s, when I was a teenager, few of us had intercourse due to fear of pregnancy as well as the taboos placed on extra-marital sex by society. However, I loved "heavy petting" and had terrific orgasms with digital stimulation and squeezing on men's thighs—or on horseback or fence railings! *(Phoebe, 64)*

Sex wasn't something you talked about unless you were telling a risqué joke. I was taught that if you slept with a guy, he'd never marry you. *(Penny, 60)*

I had missionary sex before I even heard of the phenomenon of oral sex—and then it was fellatio. My first reaction was disbelief and disgust. I'd never have thought I'd go on to consider myself an aficionada. It was years later that I heard of cunnilingus. *(Rachel, 62)*

continued on next page

continued from page 41

I came out when I was twelve years old, I think it was 1953. I was oppressed by the times, and I came from a violent family. I created my own little private world where masturbating was a way I'd feel comforted. I had my first sexual experience at fourteen with an older woman, twenty-one. I felt that was going to be my life, that I would be a sexual person. As I grew up, like many lesbians, homophobia shut me down. We were activists, and we did everything but have sex. I was considered strange for wanting to explore a sexual relationship. I had a partner say to me, "You sure like to have sex." My response was to feel ashamed. Today I would have said to her, "You know what? If sex isn't what you want to do, I need to move on." *(Claire, 66)*

I was brought up in a rural area in the 1950s, when sex was supposed to be forbidden, but several girls in my (very small) high school became pregnant. Then I had an affair with a married neighbor from age sixteen to twenty, and sex became a major focus, although I still excelled in school and got scholarships to college. My sexual experience turned out to be very valuable, both in my personal growth and as experience to draw on in my psychotherapy practice. I am very satisfied now, and no longer searching as I was. *(Tina, 61)*

When I was young, I was very affected by the abuse I suffered as a child. It wasn't horrible abuse, but I hadn't coped with the molestation even though I had a very active sex life. I was always fearful and held back. I grew up without boundaries. You don't know your own body. It belongs to someone else. I was always so confused about sex. I didn't understand what made me tighten up. *(Monica, 60)*

I was taught that sex should be saved for marriage, but that it is natural and should be enjoyed. I was never told not to masturbate or told superstitions. I was given the facts about sex whenever I asked at whatever age I asked. *(Lily, 60)*

I was raised in a very repressive environment. Everything about sex was labeled bad and forbidden. French kissing was a sin, kissing over ten seconds was a sin, masturbating was a sin. Birth control was also a sin, and so I became pregnant after my second sexual encounter at age eighteen. Although it was a scandal for an unmarried Catholic girl to be pregnant in 1965, my upbringing would not allow me to choose an abortion. Today I strongly support a woman's right to choose but have never been sorry about my choice to have the baby. My early training about sex made me quite inhibited and not very adventurous in bed. I'm sure that contributed to our marriage not lasting. It makes me angry to think about what crap I was fed as a young girl. I was careful not to continue that with my daughters. *(Susie, 60)*

I was taught that sex was something men liked and women gave to please, attract, and keep men. *(Pepper, 71)*

I was a virgin until I got married at twenty-one. In those days, we got married because that's what girls did. It was so awful for me that we couldn't even do it for two or three days. I was so small, and he was so big. We didn't even know about lubricants. The first few times we had sex, I bled all over the sheets. I don't know how these kids of today can go through that with just anybody. *(Jaime, 73)*

been for them. I wish they could have grown to have the joie de vivre that I have created in my own life, and the exhilaration of the kind of love I share with Robert.

It's True What They Say about Italian Lovers

My first really great sex was in Italy where I lived for three years after college, first on a Fulbright teaching assistantship in Modena and then as a teacher in an American private school in Florence.

Marcello, my lover for two years, was a dynamic, poetic, movie-star-handsome Florentine whose sexual understanding of women left me euphoric. He was a law student and tour guide who explained Michelangelo in three languages, recited Italian poetry to me, and spoke the language of love with his hands and with his mouth. He gloried in giving pleasure.

"Why are Italian men such good lovers?" I asked him.

"Because we understand that women want sexual pleasure even more than men, and we love giving it to them," he replied.

After Marcello broke up with me by leaving my apartment key and a brief note on my kitchen table, I had a short-lived but intense fling with Giuliano, the most sexual man I've ever known. The day of New Year's Eve, we totaled eleven orgasms between us (I don't remember how many were mine, but more than I had ever experienced before). When we finally got up and showered, and I tried to put up my hair to go out to a party, I started to faint. We never got to the party.

As I reflect now, it feels a bit odd to be equating great sex with number of orgasms. At the time, having orgasms meant that my partner was committed to my pleasure because it was physically impossible for me to achieve an orgasm just by "letting go" with the apparent ease and spontaneity that men seem to achieve. We both had to be concentrating on my special spots, using just the right motion, pressure, and pace. If I felt the man disengage emotionally—his mind wandering, or his eyes flitting to the clock, or his own urgency taking over—I was back at square one. So having an orgasm was a sort of triumph of teamwork—the two of us, in unison, made it happen.

Generation Gap?

When I was coming of age, sex was cloaked in mystery. With all the blatant sexual images and dialogue on television and in films, the language of today's music, the fashions that today's teenage girls wear, they seem much more sexually sophisticated than we were.

And yet, I recently picked up *Sex and Sensibility: 28 True Romances from the Lives of Single Women,*[1] written by young women today, and I read this account of Elissa Schappell's seventh-grade sexual curiosity: "If I started having sex, would I ever be able to stop? Was having sex like peanuts and tattoos—you couldn't have just one?"

In college, Schappell goes wild feasting at the sexual banquet, although until her senior year, she says, "I'd only been with boys who'd treated my body like some sort of finicky appliance, twisting my nipples, pressing on my clitoris as though this alone would send me into some wild and frothy spin cycle."

I laugh aloud at the realization that although in my day we didn't know that the clitoris existed, today kids might know, but they still don't know what to do with it.

Sexually Seasoned Women Compare Sex Now with Sex in Their Youth

I feel more free, adventurous, and open about what I want. As a younger woman, it was more a power trip, to see what a guy would go through to get you into bed. So often it was not as exciting as it should be. Everything that my current favorite partner does turns me on—in fact, he can't turn me off. *(Kaycee, 66)*

I'm much more appreciative of sex now. I was more interested in conquest and romance in my twenties and thirties. No worries now about getting pregnant, no concerns about how I look. As a woman, I sometimes think, *This must be what sex is like for a man.* And it's good. *(Rachel, 62)*

I love sex and always have. I seem to be attracting better men than when I was younger. My life works, I love myself, I am spiritually awakened, financially successful, and funny, nurturing, and honest. I used to be dependent on a relationship and didn't take my time selecting an appropriate partner. I just loved being mated. Now the men are better—people I totally respect. And even though they are older, they are great lovers. *(Bess, 63)*

I am much less inhibited than I was when I was younger. I feel so loved by my husband that I am no longer self-conscious about my body or any sexual activity. My husband is extremely generous and eager to please me, and I now give myself permission to just enjoy everything. *(Susie, 60)*

I used to feel dependent on someone wanting me instead of initiating anything or following my feelings and desires. It was all about pleasing my partner. Now there's no pressure to perform or prove anything. I don't worry whether it was good for him the way I used to. I'm more in control of when I want it and am more outspoken about what I want and also when I don't feel like it. Not doing it out of obligation is really good. *(Ulla, 61)*

Sex with my husband has always been good, but inhibitions, fear we'd be overheard, pregnancy concerns, and difficulty in setting aside distractions and worries were a far bigger problem then than now. I'm much less uptight. There was a time I didn't want anything to do with oral sex *(can't imagine that now!)* or sex aids. *(Mary Ann, 62)*

It is safe, steady, and regular with a man I love (my husband of two years). It's comfortable and predictable, and there's no messing around with diaphragms or worrying about pregnancy. *(Joanna, 61)*

It's different because it's calmer. It's more relaxed. You take your time. It's slower. When you're younger, it's fast. *(Matilda, 78)*

I've always felt very sexual, had lots of lovers, loved having orgasms, demanded my freedom and right to enjoyment. Generally my life is easier, less driven, so sex is a part of it rather than a driving force. It is easier not being controlled by my hormones and sex drive. Also, I feel very self-confident about my sexuality and attractiveness, pleased that I am attractive to others, even younger men. *(Phoebe, 64)*

continued on next page

continued from page 47

I have sex less than I did when I was younger, and the intensity is much less. I still enjoy sex as I did when I was younger. I don't feel like I am missing anything because of the changes as I age. Intense and frequent sex was part of my younger life, but now I am happy with the slower pace and less intensity. I don't want to go back. My sex life is satisfying. It flows into my life smoothly as I age. I am looking forward to each new year and each new decade. *(Lily, 60)*

As a young woman, I was having sex with young men. I was certainly more responsive then, but many men didn't seem to care if I had a climax or not. They finished too fast, didn't spend enough time with foreplay, and seemed unaware or unconcerned about what a women needs to finish. I only remember one man making an attempt. He held himself high with his arms so that his penis slid back and forth across my clitoris. That was great. Since women can have multiple orgasms, I wish that more men had made me climax first and then had intercourse—then maybe, just maybe, I'd have had a second orgasm during intercourse. I wish I hadn't been too timid to ask for this! I've always been open-minded, willing to try new things, but as a young woman, I found it difficult to be the initiator. *(Melanie, 64)*

Changed Expectations

I went through the first few years of my youthful sexual experience without experiencing orgasm. I didn't know how, and neither did my loving but equally inexperienced boyfriend. When I broke up with Donny at the end of my freshman year in college, for reasons unrelated to sex, I went a little wild experimenting with college boys. My first orgasm was at age nineteen, with a boy who prided himself on understanding how to "do it" using his hand before his penis. What a jolt! I even learned to do this for myself. How embarrassing that I never figured this out on my own!

Once I discovered orgasm, I celebrated it to the point that I considered any sex act when I didn't have one disappointing, unfinished, one-sided. But now, at age sixty-one, although my orgasms are intense and screamingly wonderful (Robert likened my cries to a jungle parrot, and once a neighbor thought a chicken was being killed), they're not how I measure sexual satisfaction.

I can reach euphoria with an hour of pleasuring my partner, hearing his moans, feeling his skin, and seeing his quivers. This euphoria is absolutely as intense as my own orgasm because I feel so deeply connected to this man whom I love profoundly, my dream lover. Touching, kissing, teasing, and pleasing him are ways of crawling inside his skin, melding minds, melting souls.

CHAPTER 4

The Bodies We Live In

Bloom like the Naked Lady flower. After summer the green leaves go limp, and then suddenly there's a single pink beauty standing on tiptoes and waving.
— Susan Swartz in *Juicy Tomatoes: Plain Truths, Dumb Lies, and Sisterly Advice about Life after 50*[1]

Our older bodies startle us by altering shape, weight, sensitivity, skin elasticity, moistness, hair color. We discover splotches, wrinkles, and dry spots. We feel suddenly vulnerable. And when did these aches and pains, more uninvited guests of aging, decide to set up residence inside our bodies? Rather than springing out of bed as I used to, I test the waters, inch by inch: How do my feet feel today? My back? My hip?

And yet these bodies of ours are still capable of immense pleasure and exquisite sensation. They are still our domains of delight. No, we don't live in the bodies of our youth, but our skin is still sensitive and responsive to touch, and we still open gladly to a welcome lover. I like this slogan I wear on a T-shirt: "Women have no expiration date."

> *There's nothing wrong with women's faces or*
> *bodies that social change won't cure.*
> —Naomi Wolf in *The Beauty Myth: How Images*
> *of Beauty Are Used against Women*[2]

Body Image

As a young woman in my twenties and thirties, I didn't have much trouble attracting men, especially the younger men I lusted after. I was cute, petite, assertive, and full of vitality. When I look back at photos now, I marvel that I actually worried about my hip size or unperky breasts. It's ironic and wonderful that my lover loves my widening, sixty-one-year-old hips and dimpled thighs and calls my vertically challenged breasts beautiful. I'm starting to see his viewpoint myself.

It's also ironic and wonderful that despite loose skin and the pull of gravity, I'm in much better shape than I ever was in my twenties and thirties, thanks to an ingrained exercise habit, at least three dance evenings a week, and a lover who helps me keep my body fine-tuned and responsive.

I do everything in my power to stay strong and healthy, but I'd be lying if I said I didn't care about the visual effects of aging. They surprise me every time I catch a glimpse of my sags, wrinkles, and lines. I work out, take pride in my muscles, and still go sleeveless every chance I get. But a year ago, I started to notice the lined, loose skin of my arms dominating the image in the gym mirror when I flexed my biceps. I actively choose to refocus my eyes and concentrate on the muscles that I'm keeping strong and defined.

"When you do book signings, wear a sexy camisole," Robert tells me. "Pay no attention to your wrinkly arms."

"Oh! You see my arms as wrinkly?" I wail.

"No. *You* see your arms as wrinkly," he says.

He's right. What is it about women that we have to focus on what we consider our least attractive attributes? I used to teach group exercise, and today I continue to work with a few clients as their personal trainer. Inevitably, however fit, strong, and beautiful my female clients are, they point to that one ripple, bulge, or sag—their personal archenemy.

Part of aging for me has been appreciating—even rejoicing in—the body parts that still work well, and learning to accept with humor and dignity those that don't work perfectly or look so lovely. I am aware that this is the youngest I'll be from now on.

I read quotes from my interview sources in this chapter to Robert. "Are they really all so positive about their bodies?" he asks, knowing that women in our culture seem to do everything they can to disguise or "fix"—rather than celebrate or laugh at—their bodies' signs of aging.

"They're self-selected," I tell him. "They agreed to be interviewed because they feel positive about sex, and when I asked what they loved about their bodies, everyone had a response." I'm seeing a connection: Loving and appreciating our bodies goes hand in hand with having joyful sex.

Robert Speaks about Bodies

Robert brings me coffee in bed, one of our loving rituals. I push the covers down, baring my body. "Oh, cover up!" he cries, shading his eyes, as if blinded by beauty. Though this is a game we play, I know he honestly does see my body as beautiful, and neither wrinkled skin nor dimpled buttocks interfere with his appreciation. I ask him to tell me his philosophy of finding beauty in an aging lover's body. He replies thoughtfully:

> We need to see wrinkles as attractive, wisdom as sexy. Our aesthetic appreciation of our bodies needs to change as we age, and as our lovers age, too. So much about honest sexuality at this point in our lives is not expecting to look like we're twenty-five, but living with ourselves long enough to be comfortable in our bodies, seeing beauty in older bodies, and being turned on by them. If we're not comfortable with our bodies at sixty, when will we be?
>
> When I look at you, I see the signs of your history. I see these as beautiful because they acknowledge that I am with someone who has fully lived and is fully alive. When I'm engaged in lovemaking, I become one with my lover. If

I'm concerned with being authentic—deeper than the layers of flesh—then why would I want anything other than authenticity from the woman with whom I make love?

When I look at photographs of myself, I think that I am that person with saggy jowls, straggly hair, and spotted skin. When I make love, I don't see that image. I become an energy in an ageless body. The energy—sexuality—is fluid, timeless, ageless. At orgasm, I feel one with the universe—suspended where time has no meaning. Orgasm is the big bang, the release of everything but life itself.

Our culture requires certain image upkeep. When that breaks down, or when we begin to give it up, we can either resist that change or celebrate it. There isn't much in the culture that helps us celebrate it. When was the last time we saw an older woman naked in a film without a big deal being made to point out how rare it is? Our culture bombards us with highly limiting images of body and sexuality that restrict rather than expand our responses. It's something we have to do on our own with our own maturing process.

When you made a face and your mother said, "Be careful, your face might freeze that way," she was right. It just takes longer than you think.

—Johanna Newell

Sexually Seasoned Women Speak about Their Bodies and Sexuality

I understand how gravity works. I'm aware as I position myself on top of Eric that the skin of my arms and face responds to gravity's pull downward, and I look much more wrinkled in that position than when he's on top of me. Still, our enjoyment of woman-on-top far overshadows my self-consciousness about my wrinkles, and I pretend not to realize how much older I must look in that position. *(Diana, 62)*

If the body feels good, then sex is much more a possibility. You know what? This even applies to solo sex. *(Rachel, 62)*

I have gained five pounds since not having a regular lover. I work out every day and am in great shape—but I think I am eating extra to fill the emotional hole. I love my body. I have no pain or discomfort. It is a great source of pleasure. *(Bess, 63)*

People say to me, "You look really good for sixty-seven." I say, "Don't say that!" What is that saying about my sisters? We don't like wrinkles and sags and bags. We dye our hair. Society teaches us to say, "Why should I have sex with some old, baggy person when I can have sex with someone younger?" *(Nina, 67)*

continued on next page

continued from page 55

I've always been basically critical of my own body, which is short and plump, although I do like my breasts. In honesty, I know what I think of my body is too much a reflection of what others think, or I think they think. I feel sexy with my husband because he does and always has liked my body. *(Mary Ann, 62)*

I'm a big woman, and I have nice, large breasts. Lots of times I wish I were smaller. We see these skinny women on TV, and they don't even have any thighs. I'm taking water pills, and my face looks like a prune. My lover doesn't act as if that matters. *(Bea, 77)*

I like that I am slim, and in dimmer lighting, I still appear youthful to myself. I don't like the less-than-firm state of my boobs and stomach and avoid being on top unless the lights are low. I've looked at myself in a mirror from beneath, and it's not all that attractive. *(Ulla, 61)*

I was always very self-conscious about my body. My first pregnancy, at nineteen, left me with lots of stretch marks on my stomach. After my divorce, I was always worried that a new lover would be turned off by those marks. I didn't want the lights on during lovemaking and didn't want to walk around naked. *(Susie, 60)*

I'd say I look a hell of a lot better than I ever expected to look at seventy-one. That makes me feel sexy, and I like to wear sexy nightgowns to show it off. I was unhappy with my body as I had put on ten pounds over the years. I lost the extra weight, and now I keep careful tabs on what I weigh. Right now, there isn't much I don't like about my body—just the fact that gravity is pulling its folds down more and more each year. *(Pepper, 71)*

I feel good about myself in that I take responsibility for watching my weight and keeping in shape. I want to be attractive to my partner. I don't like the wrinkles and seeing the effects of aging on my skin. *(Lily, 60)*

Yesterday I went to a pool party of mostly women. I was the only woman in a bathing suit—and I looked great in it at sixty-six—and I was the only adult who went into the very sensual hot tub and warm pool, which were full of children and preteen and teen girls. Women are so ashamed of their bodies that they can't have fun anymore. I was much like the kids, spitting water at them and playing hide and seek in the water. I was so wanting K to be there because she would have joined me and we would have sneaked a few kisses underwater. The older women sat at tables, eating and talking—yuck! Take a break, girls! *(Claire, 66)*

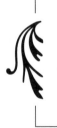

Women are not forgiven for aging. Robert Redford's lines of distinction are my old-age wrinkles.
—Jane Fonda

Facing Our Faces

I hear women ask, "When did I become my mother?" as they see their aging images. My mother died at forty-five, so I don't know what she would look like if she had lived. I know I eat healthier, exercise more, and have more joy in my life than my mother did. Has this contributed to the youthfulness I've enjoyed and protected my face from the ravages of aging, thus causing people to comment that I look younger than my age? Or is it just genes?

As a child, teenager, and young woman, I always looked much younger than I was. My size—just under five feet tall as an adult—helped, to be sure. But I also had a face that looked years younger than my chronological age.

I used to be impatient to look older because I was treated as less mature than I felt I was. Older people would tell me, "You'll be grateful that you look younger when you're my age!" Now I'm their age, and they're right. At forty I was happy to look thirty; at fifty I was elated to look fortyish.

Now, my face is catching up, and it disorients me. I inspect my face in the enlarged image of the magnifying mirror. Oh dear, the wrinkles around my lips have deepened—almost overnight, it seems—so I look like my aged French teacher in high school pursing her lips to make the "u" sound we tried so hard to mimic. I remember wondering if she knew how she looked when she did that, and whether I had to make my mouth look wizened in order to make the sounds myself.

Now I have become my French teacher, lips looking pursed even when they're relaxed. I buy special lip liner that prevents my lipstick from "bleeding" into my wrinkles. Or I go without lipstick altogether.

I wonder how freeing it would be to age in a culture that doesn't have mirrors.

I like to think that I'm the same person inside as the youthful, pretty me in the early photos—but I'm not. To twist an advertising slogan, I'm older *and* better. My experiences, my life lessons, the times I've laughed or frowned or knit my brows in puzzlement, the kisses I've given and received—they're all etched in my face. I watch young, pretty women, and I wonder who they are or will become. I watch women my age and older, and I feel a connection to who they are and what they've lived. I am amazed by their beauty.

Loving Our Labia

I can't believe this. I just got a press release about a "vaginal reconstruction expert," a surgeon who specializes in procedures such as labiaplasty—the trimming of labia minora, more commonly known as the lips of the vagina. The release reads, in part:

> *Having enlarged or irregular labia minora may adversely affect the quality of life for patients, resulting in lowered self-confidence. . . . The enlarged labia can have a protuberant and abnormal appearance that can be bothersome and*

distressful. The unsightly appearance of excessive skin can cause psychological damage and may decrease the sexual desire in both partners . . .

Great, now we're supposed to worry because our labia might be different. Guess what—we're all different. I remember being fascinated by a medical website that showed a series of women's labia. I had never seen any other woman's labia before. They were all different—shapes, colors, protuberances, and all. I can see running to a surgeon if our labia make daily life or sex uncomfortable, but please, let's not succumb to one more ridiculous beauty standard!

I ask Claire, sixty-six, her thoughts on the subject of labia beauty. She replies:

It wasn't until late in life that I began to look at my own labia, which are full and large and kind of a deep purple color. I love them because they make me feel like everything I do sexually is full, large, and deep. Once I began looking at other women's labia, I found them beautiful, like all of the parts of a woman. Who wants to be the same as the next woman anyway? I say embrace our differences and allow every woman to be beautiful in who she is.

What Color Is My Hair?

I'm in a quandary. I'm writing about aging, and how sexy we are after sixty. I work hard to keep my body strong, and I'm learning to accept what I cannot change about its wrinkles and sags. Plastic surgery isn't an option for me—it's fine for other women if they want it, but I don't want to go that direction. What you see is what I am.

Claire, Sixty-six, Learns to Love Her Hair

As I stepped out of the shower this morning and looked into the mirror, I saw my beautiful white, white hair. I started turning gray at about nineteen (it runs in my family). I dyed all the grays until I was thirty-six, when I just didn't want to deal with all the crap of dyes. It was during my process of uncovering all the shame I carried that I began to want to just be me. K loves my hair. I love my hair. I love myself finally! Oh, what a relief.

But—and this is a big but—I've been coloring my hair since gray started coming in. It feels hypocritical to dance through life with the dark brown hair of my youth, and yet a huge part of me yells, "I'm not ready!" when I think about going natural. I inspect the photos on my website—I look young and vivacious. I *feel* young and vivacious. But my hair color is fake.

I don't even know what color my natural hair would be now—an interesting, salt-and-pepper design? Dramatic silver? Soft white? Or dull gray that pulls the color out of my face and ages my appearance a decade? Isn't there a computer program that could take my face and show me wearing different permutations of gray/silver/white hair?

Robert discusses this with me non-judgmentally. As my lover, he assures me—and I believe him—that he will love me and be turned on by me whether my hair is brown or gray. As an artist, he acknowledges that I would look quite a bit older if I let my hair go natural. He supports me whichever I choose.

Robert's hair is almost pure white, soft as a cloud and just as beautiful. He likes short haircuts for the ease of maintenance, while I like his hair longer. I find his hair sensual and inviting, and I love to get my hands in it, smell the clean shampoo smell, brush my cheek or breasts against its soft texture.

I discovered men's hair in the 1960s, when they started letting it grow long. What a sensual delight! I remember the surge of arousal I felt when I removed the rubber band from Kyle's ponytail, letting his thick curls spring out around his face, inviting me to bury my hands and face in them. I remember how Richard moaned with excitement when I gently pulled his long hair during sex. I was disappointed when the style passed and men's hair went short again. I still feel a thrill when I see photos of long-haired men from that time.

Back to *my* hair. I took my problem to my hairstylist, Troy, and asked if there was a way he could start working silver (much prettier sounding than gray, don't you think?) streaks into my brown hair until I dared to go all the way gray. He thought it best to start with blond highlights to lighten things up, and then I could allow my own hair to grow in gradually. Of course, we both realized that "gradually" might mean over the next decade, not the next appointment!

I was so delighted by the look of my newly colored brown hair with blond highlights that I totally forgot it was a path to going gray. I look livelier, not older, and for now, I'll keep the look. Check in with me in a few years for an update: www .joanprice.com.

Whatever your choice about how to age—in those parts over which you *have* a choice—I support your decision. If you feel sexy with blond, black, brown, red, or purple hair, go for it.

Reclaiming My Body

Most of us learn to walk once. I've had to learn to walk from scratch three times: Once as a tot and two more times after head-on automobile accidents, sixteen years apart—both caused by out-of-control drivers.

The first nearly killed me. I suffered myriad injuries, including a smashed face, a neck fracture, and a shattered heel and ankle. The second severely fractured the leg I had rehabilitated for sixteen years. Is it any wonder that I smile when I walk and dance? I never take for granted the power of my legs to move me or the strength of my feet to bear my weight.

The first accident kept me in the hospital for almost a month, with surgeons reconstructing my face and body and painkillers taking the edge off my physical agony. I learned to hobble on crutches, one arm and one leg in a cast, my facial bones wired together, my neck positioned in a brace strapped around my chest. Although far from independent, I begged to go home. I needed to take charge of my body and my life.

"Do you have any last-minute questions?" my doctor asked as I was ready to leave the hospital.

"Yes," I replied, trying to enunciate although the wires from my facial reconstruction held my jaw clamped shut. "When can I have sex again?"

My doctor's vision slid over my broken body, focusing on my casts, brace, and wires. I could tell he was thinking, "What does she think she'll be able to do in that condition?" But he only said, "Uh, as soon as you leave here if you want—but if you move around a lot, you need to wear the neck brace."

It wasn't that I was feeling particularly sexy after that

Sexually Seasoned Women Answer the Question, "What Do You Love about Your Body?"

I have earned the wrinkles, rolls and sags, varicose veins and gray hair, and I feel blessed to be alive and healthy and to have loved and lived for sixty-four years. *(Jill, 64)*

For the first time in my life (since menopause and weight gain), I have real tits! It's true that they are flabby and somewhat saggy, but they're BIG! *(Joanna, 61)*

I love my breasts. I have gorgeous legs. I was a dancer as a younger woman, and I still feel like a dancer. I recently lost thirty pounds. I love my body. I want to start doing Pilates to tone even more. *(Barbara, 60)*

I'm overweight, but I love my body. It's been very good to me. My grandmother lived to 103, and my mother lived to 94. I'm a vegetarian, and I think I'll live a long time. *(Tina, 61)*

I think my body is great. I have all my wrinkles and brown spots, and that's fine, that's who I am. And the body works

devastating automobile accident that nearly took my life and changed it for all time. For me, after four weeks of living in a broken body that—I knew—would continue to give me challenges for the rest of my life, sex was about reclaiming my body, inviting it to provide pleasure again.

I can't say that my first sex date after leaving the hospital was

better than it ever has. The woman I'm with thinks I'm the most beautiful woman she's ever seen in her life, which makes me feel great. I wish women could just learn to love their bodies like I have done, and refuse to buy the social stuff that's out there about youth and beauty. We are all beautiful. *(Claire, 66)*

I guess my body is good for my age. I do get compliments from both men and women. I have a tummy, which bothers me, but most people don't seem to notice it. Maybe that's because I have such a big chest for such a little woman. *(Jaime, 73)*

Although when I am dressed I would like to be thinner, I feel sexy naked now. I am very curvy with large breasts, and my husband seems to delight in my body. It's not Twiggy or even fashionably thin, but I'm definitely feminine. *(Susie, 60)*

I like my skin. I've avoided the sun, so I'm still fairly wrinkle-free, and my chest and waist and stomach are fairly smooth. My breasts are small, so I don't sag too much. What I like best about my body is being touched all over. It is very pleasurable to have my lover run his hands all over my body. He says that I am a very sensuous woman. *(Melanie, 64)*

particularly exciting. My lover and I dubbed it "slug love." But it did show me that some parts still worked. Hallelujah.

Now, each time I dance or make love or just walk across a room, I feel exhilaration at having the power to move my body, to train and strengthen it, to enjoy movement for its own sake.

Fearless Women: Midlife Portraits

I am enthralled by *Fearless Women: Midlife Portraits* by writers Nancy Alspaugh and Marilyn Kentz and photographer Mary Ann Halpin.[3]

This large-format book shows powerful photographs of fifty women ages forty to sixty-plus, each posed with a sword, symbolizing courage. Some are familiar names and faces, such as Joni Mitchell, Cybill Shepherd, and Gloria Allred. Others are new to me: activists, dancers, teachers, athletes, doctors. They are all strong, self-confident women who do their work in the world and take no guff for being middle-aged.

The photos are original and beautiful, and each is placed beside a snapshot or portrait of the woman in her youth. I was startled to discover how much more beautiful these women are now. The youthful photos showed facial structure, eyes, smiles—but none of the complexity of a woman's face as it begins to reflect her experience, her history, her wisdom. Looking at these fifty women, I imagine my own photo among them.

How would I look now, a current photograph beside the air-brushed portrait from my sophomore year in college? I wore a complex, bouffant hairstyle—teased hair in a French twist—and the only lines on my face were drawn in with liquid eyeliner. I

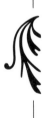

There is more wisdom in your body than in your deepest philosophy.
—Friedrich Nietzsche

guess the early photo is pretty, but I remember how confused I was about my identity, my purpose in life, my sexuality, my future. My smile was as posed as my hands. I had just broken up with my first love and had several unsatisfying flings, and didn't have a clue who I was—or who I would become.

Yes, I prefer my wrinkles.

CHAPTER 5

It Ain't Easy
after Menopause

There will be sex after death, we just won't be able to feel it.
—Lily Tomlin

In my mid-fifties, after four years of post-menopausal celibacy, I developed a relationship with a new man. During our first sexual encounters, my labia and vaginal tissues tore—little lesions bled and burned, despite using lubricant. This wasn't rough sex—it was getting-to-know-you, sweet sex with a new lover, but my labia and vagina had become thin-skinned and dry through hormone depletion and disuse. I was devastated. Were these my genitals, formerly the reliable and indestructible fountain of pleasure?

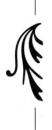

Women can now expect to live an average of eighty-two years, which means that women will now live one-third of their lives postmenopausally.
—Sheryl A. Kingsberg, PhD[1]

Post-Menopausal Angst: Has My Sex Life Ended?

No, no, no, we're not retreating now! We were the bold settlers of the new sexual frontier. Many of us threw off our clothing along with the should-nots our parents and society tried to instill in us, while the world watched. Now we have a new frontier to explore: sexual vitality after age sixty, seventy, and why not eighty? Let's set up camp and work out solutions—as we women have always done so successfully.

We're offended by outdated stereotypes of asexual older women, and we're not going to hide behind them at this time of our lives. Specifically, we're not going to roll over and play dead when our private parts are concerned. Admittedly, there are problems with sex after menopause, but we can adjust to our post-menopausal changes without losing our sexy zest.

Sexually Seasoned Women Speak about Post-Menopausal Challenges

My sexual appetite definitely cooled down after menopause, and it was more difficult to have an orgasm. I would enjoy the lovemaking but not climax. I didn't want to discourage my husband, so I would fake it a lot. I also experienced some vaginal dryness and tenderness so that intercourse was a bit painful, especially if it had been more than a couple of days since we made love. These symptoms were worse when I stopped taking hormone replacement therapy. Being tired is more of a problem than it used to be. I try to get my husband to bed by 10:30 if I want to have sex. By midnight, I'd rather sleep. *(Susie, 60)*

Hot flashes kept me up a lot at night, and I couldn't cuddle like I did before. I'd go off HRT for a while, but when the hot flashes got bad, I'd go back on. I also used wet scarves, rags, fans, and herbal supplements, but only the hormones curtailed the hot flashes. I tried natural hor-

Whew, That's Over

I remember how amazed I was at perimenopause. My periods went from regulated rain to nonstop torrents and finally to unpredictable drizzles. I had headaches that lasted three days. My mood swings walloped me incessantly, imprisoning me in an emotional boxing ring. I was glad I lived alone.

I didn't really mind the hot flashes—despite my histrionics in "The Boomers Approach Menopause (Kicking and Scream-

mone replacement, but that didn't really help. I finally went off everything three years ago. I still have hot flashes. Not as much as before, but they still keep me from spooning as contact sets them off. *(Lily, 60)*

Early menopause coincided with my separation and divorce from my first partner and meeting and shacking up with a new long-term partner. I can't tell what came first, the chicken or the egg. The only challenge was dryness after I stopped taking estrogen/progesterone, which I had taken for ten to fifteen years post-menopause. It took a long time to get comfortable with—and unembarrassed by—the pause to apply K-Y Jelly. My partner helped by being the one to stop and apply it instead of my having to initiate the act. *(Pepper, 71)*

I don't always experience orgasm, and it's sometimes challenging to go back to it later to bring it to completion. I want a more loving, holding, and caressing type of lovemaking and less "doing it." Cuddling and emotional, nurturing parts of lovemaking are almost more important than actual intercourse, although it's nice to end that way. *(Ulla, 61)*

ing)" (see sidebar "Hot Flash Flashbacks" on next page). I found simple ways to cope. I taught aerobics with an ice-filled water bottle stuck in my leotard top, held snugly between my breasts and the Lycra as I danced, stepped, and lifted weights. I bought a little plastic, battery-operated fan that I carried around and aimed strategically. I didn't heat my house for two years (my few guests didn't remove their coats and gloves when they visited me in the winter).

Hot Flash Flashbacks

The following was excerpted from an article I wrote for the *Pacific Sun* in 1994 called "The Boomers Approach Menopause (Kicking and Screaming)"[2]

The fashion industry doesn't have a clue what the Boomer female wants. Forget Wonderbras! Give us a line of "Hot Flash Wear"! I want a shirt made of large patches attached with Velcro. When the flash hits and my skin feels like an electric blanket gone amok, I rip the patches open and cool my dermatological hotspots. When it subsides, I slap the patches back on.

I've seen boxer shorts with condom pockets advertised for the twenty-something guys. Where are the quick-zip-down-the-front, scoop-neck blouses with oriental-fan pockets for us menopausal gals?

Whew, got that off my sweaty chest.

I am fifty and going through menopause. I always figured if I ate a nutritious, low-fat diet, eschewed unhealthy habits, and exercised my buns off, I'd get through the transition unscathed. I'm still holding onto that thought, but goodness, the experience is more powerful than I anticipated!

Hot flashes strike night and day. My inner furnace blasts unpredictably while I'm eating, sleeping, making love, writing (here comes one now), or teaching aerobics. I can be high on life one minute and in tears the next.

And the . . . uh . . . er . . . oh, yeah, memory loss! I spend ten minutes looking for my purse (it's on my shoulder) or my keys (in the door I just opened). Hint: Never, never move something a menopausal woman has put somewhere and spent good brainpower memorizing!

A generation ago, women didn't talk about menopause. We're talking up a storm now. At parties, in gym locker rooms, at coffee breaks, we're discussing hot flashes, urine leaks, and vaginal dryness with as little embarrassment as we once compared diets, men, or childrearing techniques. We're hungry for information.

Our talk boils down to three major concerns: 1. "Is [insert symptom] a normal symptom of menopause?" 2. "Should I go on hormone replacement therapy?" and 3. "What natural/alternative therapies are effective?"

The answer to Number One is pretty simple—usually "yes" will suffice. Symptoms may be subtle, or they may feel like PMS on steroids. They may include any assortment of hot flashes, anxiety, night sweats, insomnia, irritability, joint pain, bloating, constipation, mood swings, headaches, urinary tract problems, or a number of other imbalances. The onslaught of symptoms may appear not with the cessation of menstruation but for a sometimes multiyear phase preceding menopause.

The answers to Numbers Two and Three, we're finding, are far from clear-cut.

I welcomed menopause—no more PMS, no more bloating, no more boxes of tampons (light, medium, heavy) under the sink and in my purse, no more panic when my period didn't arrive on schedule, no more rinsing underwear in cold water, no more bloody sheets, no more fear of wearing white. (My hip spread eliminated white from my lower half's wardrobe anyway, but that's another story.) Some women feel like menopause is an ending—I felt it was a new beginning.

Hormone Hubbub: Our Generation's Dilemma

"Don't take away my HRT!" a zesty, Boomer-aged woman pleads with her doctor. That's the problem—many of us feel better, younger, sexier with HRT. Yet we can't—shouldn't—ignore the studies that are getting pounded into our minds that show for most of us, the risks probably outweigh the benefits. We're all different, and we can't know for sure whether, in our individual case, HRT is good for us or bad for us, and which type/combination/brand might be better or worse.

The medical evidence that came to light in 2002 was frightening enough to make many of us throw away our pills. Yes, HRT stops hot flashes and keeps our vaginal tissues from thinning, and it seems to lower the risk of colorectal cancer and bone fractures. But it seems to increase the risk of breast cancer. And whoops, we thought it reduced the risk of heart disease, but actually it increases this risk, along with the risk of strokes and blood clots.

Boomers are the experimental generation. Our doctors put us on HRT, then new studies come out and we go off, or try alternatives. Is it estrogen or progesterone or the combination that increases risk? Does natural progesterone make a difference? Is the estrogen patch better than the pill? How about a lower dose? Or the estrogen ring? Or estrogen cream? In another twenty years, I'll bet medical science will know exactly who should or should not go on HRT after menopause, and what kind, when, for how long, why, and why not. But for now, we make our best guesses.

Melanie's HRT Story

Melanie, sixty-four, voices the concerns of many postmenopausal women trying to reconcile their emotional desire for sex with their diminishing physical sensitivity:

> *I really, really miss my HRT.*
>
> *Hormone replacement therapy worked great for me for fifteen years. I could make myself climax in less than a minute with my vibrator. I would rest just a bit and then continue. I could climax over and over.*
>
> *I ignored the warnings that came out about heart problems, but when they mentioned dementia, I was afraid.*
>
> *I quit taking HRT just about the time I met my current boyfriend. I definitely can tell that there has been a tapering off of my sexual sensitivity. I just don't have the tingling or nearly as much sensitivity as before. If we decide that I would like to come, we get out the vibrator. And it usually takes some time now, even with the vibrator.*

Ice, Pills, Patches, Creams, and Rings

Since I wrote "The Boomers Approach Menopause (Kicking and Screaming)" (see sidebar "Hot Flash Flashbacks on pages 72–73") more than ten years ago, the decision whether or not to stay on HRT

Sexually Seasoned Women Speak about HRT and Alternatives

I took estrogen for years and then stopped using it when everyone got nervous about estrogen. I started having hot flashes again at sixty-five. When my libido flagged even though I was in this great relationship, I started using testosterone. I think I've noticed a feeling of arousal, and I grab my vibrator and have an orgasm. *(Nina, 67)*

I had a total hysterectomy at age forty-seven and went into sudden, difficult menopause—hot flashes, no sexual responsiveness. I started Premarin, and that made a big, but not total, difference. But when all the negative research findings came out, I gradually weaned myself off Premarin and did lose some sexual responsiveness. *(Tana, 60)*

After stopping HRT, I got an estrogen ring to add a small amount of estrogen to the vagina. It works wonderfully. The dryness and tenderness greatly improved. My pubic hair is thicker again, too. There was still some discomfort, but a bit of topical estrogen cream helps that. I bought a vibrator through the mail, the one that Dr. Ruth recommends, and it has been a great help to orgasm. My husband likes it, too. The greatest help is marijuana. I am certain that the reason the United States government is so irrational about pot is that it would put Viagra and other drugs out of business. A puff or two is enough for a really fantastic sexual experience. *(Susie, 60)*

Avlimil, which my nurse practitioner recommended, is a soy product with black cohosh and other herbs and things. I've only been taking it for a month, and I do believe it is helping because I surprised myself by climaxing the last time I had sex with my boyfriend. I wasn't expecting it because I wasn't even using the vibrator! *(Melanie, 64)*

I take 0.5 milligrams of estrogen daily, which is safer for me than for many other women because I had a hysterectomy. The estrogen helps with lubrication, vaginal wall fragility, and other elements of aging. *(Mary Ann, 62)*

I so looked forward to menopause that when it happened I was thrilled. I never had a problem, not even one hot flash. Menopause was my friend. I took wild yam root capsules every day, and I had no symptoms. *(Catherine, 65)*

I took HRT specifically because I didn't want to lose my sexual drive, and I'm still taking low-dose estrogen and progesterone. I went through a difficult time when my mother died, and then when my husband was diagnosed with cancer. It's hard to tell what was hormones and what was just life. *(Tina, 61)*

After menopause, only vaginal dryness concerned me. I tried using estrogen suppositories but didn't like those, so I ended up with an Estring (estrogen ring), which my doctor prescribed. I like it a lot because I am lubricated all the time. Sometimes I can't orgasm as often as I'd like, but my husband always can, and that is very satisfying to me. I enjoy the physical contact almost as much as an orgasm. *(Penny, 60)*

has become even murkier. At the time I was going through meno-pause, we thought that hormone replacement therapy protected against heart disease, and I had a family history of heart disease. I had a bone scan and was discovered to have osteopenia, the pre-liminary stage of thinning bones. I went on traditional HRT.

When the next wave of studies started coming out, I tried variations of HRT to try to maximize the benefits and mini-mize the risks, guided by my gifted nurse practitioner, who stayed abreast of the research. I tried estrogen cream but found it too messy. (After all, oral sex is one of life's great pleasures.) For several years, I settled on the estrogen patch plus progester-one. Then I switched to a lower-dose patch, then combined it with natural instead of synthetic progesterone, and finally gave up the patch and progesterone entirely because the new medical reports were too convincing.

When Robert and I fell in love, I was surprised and disoriented by the changes in my physical responses. I was madly in love with this man, and as emotionally charged as a teenager at the thought of making love with him. So why were my physical sensations lag-ging behind my emotional excitement? Yes, I could reach orgasm, but it took a long time. (See Chapter 8, "Beds Afire: Stoking the Slower-Burning Flame," for the nitty-gritty details.) My nurse practitioner recommended a lab test for testosterone level. This male hormone is also instrumental in female sexual response.

Yes, indeed, my testosterone level was way below normal. I got a prescription for testosterone cream, to be inserted vagi-nally. We didn't know for sure how much I should take. Try this amount, have another lab test. Still too low? Try this amount. Wow, way too high now, decrease. It was messy stuff, and I had to

Important Disclaimer

This is not a medical book, and anecdotal information should never be confused with scientific proof that something works. Even if something does work for one woman, that doesn't mean it will work for you, or that it won't have undesirable side effects or interact with a medication you take in a way you don't expect. Please consult your own healthcare provider to find the best medical or alternative solution for you. Tell your doctor about any herbs or supplements you are taking. Do not take any anecdotes here as medical advice.

be sure to use it when we were not going to be having sex (which means when we weren't going to be together), but close enough that the effects lasted. The effects were negligible anyway—sometimes I thought sensation increased, but the next time it didn't. Robert hated it, especially after I started to develop facial hair. That was enough—I didn't renew the prescription.

Robert reassured me that I was just fine in my natural state, and he didn't care how much foreplay I needed to get aroused—he was happy to make love to me all afternoon.

We all need to make our own decisions about HRT and alternatives, and what to do about the effects of dwindling hormone levels. For now, I'm happy using only an estrogen ring internally to thicken the vaginal skin so I don't tear, and lubricant for comfort during sex. My nurse practitioner tells me the effects of the ring are local and are thought not to affect the rest of the body. I hope the next studies don't refute that.

Painful Intercourse Problem-Solving

By Ellen Barnard, MSSW, and Molly Webb

Painful intercourse due to vaginal dryness and vaginal atrophy can be helped by using a combination of massage (to bring healthy blood to your tissue), Liquid Silk (to moisturize your tissue), and a silicone-based lubricant like Eros (to seal the moisture into your tissue and provide a slippery surface).

Many women experience vaginal dryness—whether it's the result of menopause, prescription medications, medical conditions, or just how you are. Using lubricant during sexual activity can greatly increase your comfort level and prevent tearing, friction burns, and painful intercourse.

1. To get your sensitive tissues ready for comfortable, consensual sexual activity, start by making genital massage a part of your foreplay. You or your partner can gently massage the pubic mound (the part covered by pubic hair), inner and outer labia, clitoral hood, and clitoris. You may notice your genitals starting to turn pink or light red—this is caused by fresh blood being brought closer to the surface.

2. Next, incorporate Liquid Silk lubricant into the massage. You or your partner can use a quarter-sized amount and rub the lubricant gently into the labia, clitoris, clitoral hood, and as far into the vagina as possible. Think of Liquid Silk as a lotion for your genitals—the same way you put hand lotion on when your hands are dry, you can gently massage Liquid Silk into the genital skin to moisturize the tissues and prevent dryness.

3. Once the Liquid Silk is slightly absorbed into your skin (and you and your partner are nice and aroused!),

apply a silicone-based lubricant like Eros. Silicone-based lubricants do not soak into your skin but rather sit on the surface and provide a very slippery feeling. Applying the silicone lubricant on top of the Liquid Silk seals in the moisture the Liquid Silk brings to your skin, and also provides a layer of protection for your genital skin.

If you choose to have intercourse, this three-step process will help ensure that your genital tissue is full of fresh, healthy blood, moisturized, protected, and slippery!

If you experience pain even after trying this approach, we recommend adding a couple more steps:

4. Use Liquid Silk along with a five-minute massage of your labia, the opening of the vagina, and the outer part of the vagina every day. Gently massage the Liquid Silk into the skin, pressing down and moving your finger in a small circle, not rubbing in long strokes. You can use a small vibrator to help do this deeper into the vagina if you like. We also suggest getting a slim vibrator, covering it with lubricant, inserting it into the vagina, and letting it run for five minutes—it does the massaging for you where your fingers cannot reach.

5. Do your Kegels daily, with a focus on the end of the exercise, which should include conscious relaxation and a deep breath after each contraction. This helps you gain flexibility and learn to relax your pelvic floor muscles more consciously so you can relax during penetration.

Ellen Barnard, MSSW, is a sex educator, activist, and co-owner of A Woman's Touch Sexuality Resource Center in Madison, Wisconsin (www.a-womans-touch.com). Molly Webb is a pleasure specialist for A Woman's Touch.[3]

Juicy is an attitude, I've come to realize, based not on the flow of our vaginal secretions but on physical well-being, emotional state, mental attitude, and love of sex. Here's to post-menopausal zest—and understanding lovers!

CHAPTER 6

Fitness and Exercise: Our Bodies, Ourselves, Our Sex Lives

Keeping your blood vessels flexible helps keep your sexual arousal alive. It's also easier to achieve orgasm when blood flow to the whole body is healthy. It's as easy as walking at a moderate pace for thirty minutes a day. Take the stairs when you can during the day, or do your armchair push-ups. Rev your engine regularly!

—Myrtle Wilhite, MD[1]

Sex isn't just what we and our partners do together, and it surely doesn't reside in the genitals exclusively. Women who have great sex at any age are comfortable in their bodies and appreciate how they look and feel. Our bodies are where we live! Fitness isn't body weight or shape—it's simply being physically active as part of our lifestyle.

Exercise has the wonderful health and fitness benefits of making me the best I can be—and it also makes me feel sexier. It's partly the increased blood flow, which goes to my genitals as well as my brain and other body parts. It's also the pure physicality, which focuses my attention on my body and on bodies in general. I'm stronger, more limber, more energetic, and more in tune with my body because I exercise. This is something I do for myself that puts a zing in all parts of my life.

Body in Motion

Exercise makes you a better and more enthusiastic lover. With regular physical activity, you'll feel more vital and energetic, all your systems will function better, and you'll feel better about your appearance. An exercise habit has many health benefits—we all know that—and it also enhances sexual pleasure in these ways:

- Revs up energy
- Increases endurance
- Increases blood flow to genitals
- Decreases stress
- Lifts mood
- Improves body image and enjoyment of own body and partner's body
- Increases comfort during extended sex in various positions

- Raises levels of testosterone, the hormone that controls libido in women as well as men
- Improves self-image
- Enhances feelings of well-being
- Promotes sexy feelings

Get Physical Together

Making physical activity part of your routine with your partner has the additional benefit of making you feel closer in a physical way before you start stripping. A workout becomes foreplay when you engage in it together. Robert and I love to take country walks together, talking and laughing, admiring nature, and feeling our muscles strengthen and our stress dissipate with every stride.

I had a lover in the past who was as much into working out at the gym as I was. We often did our strength-training routines together, appreciating each other's pumped muscles, getting turned on by the intense body focus and by exercising in skimpy attire. I noticed how our flushed faces and sweat-glossed skin resembled our appearance during sex, and this turned me on. So did touching the strong, contoured muscles later.

You might enjoy a yoga class together, or a bike ride, or a gym workout. My favorite physical activity with a partner (well, second favorite) is dancing. You can choose a form of dance that's sexy and sultry, like tango or rumba; sexy and fast, like salsa; or sexy and romantic, like waltz or nightclub two-step. Any kind of dance can put you in the mood, just because it's so physical. (See Chapter 7, "Public Sex Acts and Private Preparations," for more on dancing as foreplay.)

Sexually Seasoned Women Speak about Exercise That Makes Them Feel Sexy

Swimming, especially in the nude, is very sensual and leaves me feeling sexy. *(Susie, 60)*

I try to do aerobics and weight lifting for an hour a day, three days a week. It keeps my legs tight, my arms fairly taut, my torso not sagging. We dance rarely but still love it when we do, and we know we look good together when we dance. *(Pepper, 71)*

I'm athletic, and I stay in shape. I do some yoga in the morning. I use hand weights. I ride my bike almost daily. I stopped eating junk when my cancer was diagnosed. I want to look good. I want to look sexy. *(Claire, 66)*

I exercise regularly and try to keep toned. I can dance for three hours straight and not get tired. I have good

Researchers Say . . .

• Women are more sexually responsive following twenty minutes of vigorous exercise, according to female sexuality researcher Cindy Meston, PhD, assistant professor of clinical psychology at the University of Texas at Austin. Their bodies respond to sexual arousal more quickly and intensely than when they haven't exercised.[2]

• Individuals who exercise regularly feel better about themselves, perceive they are more sexually desirable, and experience

stamina. I value my health. It enables me to enjoy life and sex. *(Melanie, 64)*

I work out three times a week. My body looks better now than it has in at least ten years. I have so much energy, and I think my confidence level is at an all-time high. Feeling physically fit adds so much to my sexuality. *(Kaycee, 66)*

I exercise regularly and dance often. These two things are key to my feeling good about myself, and because they keep me in good shape, they definitely contribute to making me feel desirable. I see my body aging, but I am still in pretty great shape for sixty. I have a lot of energy and feel good about my body. It makes me feel sexy to know that my husband thinks I have a great butt! *(Penny, 60)*

I walk almost every day and go to the gym a couple of times a week. When I'm traveling, which is frequently, I walk a lot. Also I swim whenever I can. When I exercise, I feel and look better. *(Phoebe, 64)*

greater levels of satisfaction, according to the *Electronic Journal of Human Sexuality*.[3]

• Tell the man in your life that exercise staves off erectile dysfunction! Men who started to exercise in midlife had a 70 percent reduced risk for erectile dysfunction compared to sedentary men, according to a study reported in the *Journal of the American Medical Association*. And they didn't have to run marathons, either—the equivalent of a daily two-mile brisk walk was enough.[4]

Exercise to Get the Tingle Started

Want to get in the mood on your own? Try the Pelvic Rock: Lie on your back, knees bent, feet flat on floor. Gently rock your pelvis up (off the floor a few inches) and down (returning to the floor) while squeezing your pelvic floor muscles (the Kegel muscles). You can also do this seated, rocking back and forth in your chair. Repeat five to ten times, or until you're tempted to grab your vibrator or partner.

Exercises to Enhance Horizontal Workouts

Strengthening particular muscles can make sex more pleasurable or comfortable and let you last longer without fatigue. Some mimic positions or actions you do during sex. Here are a few of my favorites:

Elevated Pelvic Rock with Squeeze: Lie on your back, knees bent, feet flat on the floor. Contract your pelvic floor muscles first, then your buttocks, as you press into your feet, lifting your lower body off the floor. From this position, rock your pelvis and do your Kegels, without lowering to the floor. (You'll be in a hammock position at the lower point, a bridge position at the top.)

Inner Thigh Clench: Lie on your back, legs in the air and slightly apart. Place your arms against your inner thighs and try to push your legs apart. Resist with the legs pressing against the arms, trying to push your arms together. Alternate letting the thighs win (the arms come together), then letting the arms win (the thighs open), and repeat. (Variation: you can squeeze a fitness ball or beach ball between your thighs and let your arms rest.)

Inner Thigh Stretch: Flexibility is as important as strength for the inner thighs, so that they can open comfortably to receive your lover. Lie on your back, legs in the air, and let your legs open out to a comfortable position. Keep your abdominal muscles engaged so that your back doesn't arch. Relax, breathing deeply. On each exhalation, let your legs open a little more. Never force or bounce when you stretch—just relax, and let the stretch happen gently. You'll find that over time, your flexibility will increase.

Quad Strengtheners: Kneel on a cushioned surface (bed or mat). Fall backward a few inches, keeping your abs tight and your body in a straight line from knees to head, then straighten up by tightening your thighs and buttocks. Repeat, each time falling back just a little more. The muscles in the front of the thighs come in handy when you're on top and sitting straight up to give your partner a lovely show.

Hip Circles: Stand with knees slightly bent and circle your hips, as if you were trying to keep a hula hoop (remember those?) in the air. Play with the movement, sometimes making large, slow circles, sometimes tight, fast circles.

Bent-Leg Push-Ups: If you like to be on top, strengthening your chest and arm muscles will help you stay there without fatiguing. Start on your hands and knees. Lift your chest, roll your hips forward, and straighten your body into a line from head to knees—this is your starting position. Bend your elbows to lower your body, leading with your chest (not your chin). Keep your abdominals tight—no sagging hips. Straighten your arms to push up. Do this exercise slowly to develop strength.

Abs Anytime, Anywhere: Feel better about yourself when

you're on top (and keep your back supported) by practicing keeping your abdominals pulled in all the time, whatever else you're doing.

Kegels Anytime, Anywhere: Do your Kegels throughout the day, wherever you are, anytime you think about it. You can do them while you're riding in a car, sitting at the computer, reading the newspaper, stirring soup on the stove—anytime you're sitting, standing, or lying down. For a real charge, do them with your partner's fingers or penis inside you!

Zip Up Your Pelvic Floor

"Learn where your pelvic floor is—and learn how to exercise it," suggests Myrtle Wilhite, MD, MS, and co-owner of A Woman's Touch Sexuality Resource Center in Madison, Wisconsin. "Tension of the pelvic floor is critical to most people's experience of feeling turned on," she explains. "When pelvic floor strength starts to slip—which is accelerated by loss of estrogen—you may begin to feel as though nothing happens down there any more."

We've all been told how to do Kegels: Squeeze on the muscles you would use to stop the flow of urine, and work up to doing lots of them fast. But that's incorrect and won't give you the real benefits, according to Dr. Wilhite. The urine-stopping muscles are just the two or three smallest of the six pelvic floor muscles, leaving the largest muscles "behind"—pun intended. And doing lots of fast Kegels fatigues these muscles without strengthening them properly.

"The pelvic floor muscles are slow-to-contract muscles, and what Kegels aim for is the resting tone of the muscles," says Dr.

Wilhite. It's far better to do just five to ten complete Kegels, contracting and then relaxing the entire pelvic floor slowly.

Here are Dr. Wilhite's instructions for one perfect Kegel:

1. First, sit on your fingertips, with the tips pointing at each other, and the fingertip pads placed right on your sits bones. Over your fingertips are your butt muscles, and those should stay nice and soft (un-contracted). Between your fingertips is the area of your pelvic floor, but up a bit, inside of your body.

2. Begin by contracting the muscles "in front" around your urethra and clitoris (the shaft and legs, really). Then, thinking of a zipper, hold onto those muscles and "zip" a little further back.

3. Then move to the third zip back.

4. Then the fourth. (You're still holding onto the first ones, just like a zipper.)

5. Then the fifth.

6. Finally, zip all the way back to your tailbone. Now your whole pelvic floor is "zipped."

7. Release all of the muscles at the same time.

8. Take a deep breath. Notice that all of the muscles relax just that bit more—those were the involuntary muscles relaxing.

All that is one Kegel! Now, get off of your fingertips before they lose circulation. The point of sitting on your fingers is just to make sure your butt muscles never clench. Once you've learned that, you don't have to sit on your fingers any more.

Five to ten of those Kegels is more than enough in one session, and two sessions per day is ideal. No need to do more because you'd be fatiguing the muscles rather than strengthening them.[5]

Strength Training My Sex Muscles

I'm a fitness professional, with a home studio full of exercise paraphernalia. So of course I took Dr. Wilhite's suggestion and obtained two tools designed specifically for training my pelvic floor muscles from www.a-womans-touch.com:

Energie Exerciser: This coated metal exerciser/stimulator weighs one pound, three ounces and measures six and a half inches long by one and a quarter inches wide at its widest point. Insert it into the vagina and leave it there while doing your Kegels and stimulating your clitoris at the same time. The rocking sensation will kindle your internal hot spots.

Stone Exercise Egg: The Crystal Stone Egg is a pelvic floor strength trainer, about two inches long by one and a half inches wide. You can insert it to do your Kegels, during self-stimulation, and for Tantric sexual massage exercises. You can even wear it for stimulation while walking, dancing, or rocking in a rocking chair. For added resistance, if you want to challenge the muscles, you can tie the storage bag to the string of the Egg and put coins in the bag to increase the weight. (Better not wear it in public this way—it would be difficult to explain if you, pardon the pun, laid an Egg!)

Pilates for Great Sex

"Make the move strong and juicy. Make it come from the hips."

No, I'm not getting instruction for acting in a porn film, nor am I rehearsing for a cabaret dance show. Chantill Lopez, my Pilates instructor, is guiding me through a training session.

I had been an exerciser for almost thirty years before I took a serious look at Pilates, although it has been around for more than eighty years. It intrigued me and offered me new fitness challenges that felt like a good direction for me, especially because I had been diagnosed with the early stages of osteoporosis. Adding Pilates to my personal exercise program helps me strengthen my core muscles for balance and posture, protect the spine, and improve my dancing. I had no idea how much I'd love it, or how sexy it would make me feel.

I was delighted to discover that in addition to all the strengthening and flexibility benefits, Pilates made me feel downright sexy! Of course, it didn't take much to make me feel sexy since I was happily in an exciting, new relationship with the man of my dreams, but even so, I have to give Pilates credit for some of the new vitality and muscle integration that I started to feel.

Pilates emphasizes core training—deep, powerful use of abdominal and back muscles—and making every movement—arm, thigh, shoulder—come from the core. Pilates teaches the balance of mobilization and stabilization, and how to make all our body parts work together like a fine-tuned, precision machine.

How does this translate to sex? I've felt sexier since I started a serious Pilates practice. I stand straighter, and I feel stronger and more balanced—physically and emotionally. I'm discovering that keeping my core stabilized and other muscles relaxed where I usually tighten out of habit and stress (neck and shoulders, for example), I can last longer without muscle fatigue and enjoy myself more. Also, the pelvic floor muscles are an integral part of the core, and I can feel them strengthening as I work through my Pilates exercises. My abs, inner thighs, and back are stronger, and my hips are more flexible. Feels good.

Ginger: Pilates Revs Up Sex

Although Ginger is only thirty-nine, she describes the bedroom benefits of Pilates so well that I had to relax my "sixty or better" age rule to share this with you:

I first heard about the positive bedroom effects on a television special with the Dixie Chicks. Natalie Maines, the lead singer, mentioned that the bandmates bring a Pilates trainer and equipment on the road with them. She talked briefly about how they loved Pilates and how the strength building really helped for stamina while touring. Then she said, "And it can do wonders for your sex life. I'm having the best sex of my life!"

I asked my husband if he noticed anything different after I had been doing Pilates for about six months. He said that everything felt more snug, and, yes, it was better for him.

As I've continued to progress with Pilates, I have noticed how the core strength has increased in my thighs, sacrum, gluteus, pelvic muscles, and abdominals. All of this really helps me get into and stay in positions that let my husband penetrate more deeply, and I can adjust things as we go along and increase the sensations as I focus on various muscles.

I can also feel my husband inside me in a way I didn't before, inch by inch, as we make love. Each time we have sex, I feel a new place inside my body. We both enjoy ourselves more because nothing is humdrum—there are always new sensations. My orgasms are definitely longer and stronger—I feel them deep and internal.

Tina Turner, at sixty-five, credits Pilates for keeping her in shape—though I'll bet her dancing and DNA play a part, too.

Go Get Sexy

You can get a great workout without setting foot in a gym, and you can learn sensual skills and get fit at the same time. I sampled these sexy workouts while researching an article for the *Pacific Sun* in Marin County, California:

Belly Dance: I've spent the last forty years wishing my belly and hips were smaller, so it is with some trepidation that I decide to let them dance and undulate at WorldDance Fitness in San Anselmo (www.worlddancefitness.com). "Belly dance is primal and spiritual, deeply feminine," co-owner and belly dance instructor Aruna tells me. "You can have hips—if you don't, we decorate them to look bigger." Where else do you get that in this culture?

Pole Dance: Butt out, chest out, look over shoulder, hip out, wrap leg around pole, swing—I never realized that pole dancing would require such strength and coordination. This sensual workout at Stage Dor Studio in Sausalito (www.stagedor.com) is much more than slithering around a pole—it strengthens the upper body (sometimes your arms are holding your whole body weight on the pole) and feels delightfully sensuous. Yes, we used a real pole. (No, we didn't strip.)

Theatrical Burlesque: I strut, shimmy, and chair dance, a feather boa flipped over my black lace camisole and push-up bra. Whatever your age, shape, size, or, uh, experience, you can be a burlesque queen for an hour in Stage Dor's sexy, mood-lifting class. "I'm not a young, tall, thin blonde," a sixty-plus fellow exerciser in a provocative, short, black dress and big, silver earrings tells me. "We all have our own brand of sexiness."

If you like the idea of finding a sexy workout or practicing sensual moves you can use to delight your partner but you'd rather do it in private, try a video such as Erotic Strip Dance (which can be purchased on www.a-womans-touch.com), Urban Striptease Aerobics (www.urbanstriptease.com), or The Art of Exotic Dancing for Everyday Women (www.artofexoticdancing.com).

Choosing a Workout That Works for You

Surprise: I was never a physically active child or young adult, didn't even learn to ride a bicycle until age twenty-six. I loved to dance as a teenager, though, and in my early thirties, I discovered aerobic dance. What a high—literally! I latched onto an everyday exercise habit just because I loved aerobic dance.

Now I love social dancing, especially contemporary line dancing. My usual weekly fitness routine includes two weight-training sessions, two Pilates sessions, as much walking as I can fit in, and about eight to ten hours of line dancing and partner dancing. None of this is grueling—it's a highlight of my day. It makes me feel good, it's good for me, and I love it. (You'd think I was talking about sex!)

That's the key—you gotta love it, or you won't stick to it. As a fitness professional, my motto is, "Exercise should be a treat, not a treatment," and I help my clients discover the fitness program that will work for them because they enjoy it, it fits their schedule and lifestyle, and it gets them to their goals.

If you think you're too busy to set aside time to exercise, you might find that daily life exercise works best for you—

simply getting more active in the way you run your life and working physical activity into your daily routine. My book, *The Anytime, Anywhere Exercise Book: 300+ Quick and Easy Exercises You Can Do Whenever You Want!*, is a collection of quickie fitness activities you can do wherever you are, whatever else you're doing—at work, at home, in a hotel, while watching television, even in an airport.

Lest you scoff at the idea of the benefits of "fitness minutes," a recent National Institutes of Health study found that subjects who engaged in "lifestyle activity" lost as much weight as high-intensity aerobic exercisers, and were more likely to maintain their fitness improvements a year later.

Your fitness choice doesn't have to be a gym workout—though it might be, if you enjoy it. Depending on your schedule and preferences, you might want to take a yoga class or hike or swim. Or you might enjoy social exercise: walks or bike rides with friends or social dancing, for example. My fitness books are full of suggestions. (See my website, www.joanprice.com, for information about my books about exercise. Tell me you're a reader of this book, and I'll give you a discount.)

CHAPTER 7

Public Sex Acts and Private Preparations

Most of sex is psychological—most of it is between our ears and not between our legs.

—Joy Browne, psychologist and radio talk-show host

Sex, for me, starts long before we get naked and continues after we get naked but before our genitals get in the act. What we do in public, in private, and with or without each other to heat up and establish intimacy in advance can make the difference between lukewarm and really hot sex.

Anytime, Anywhere: Starting Sex before Bed

I park in Robert's driveway, greeted by the bright colors of his freshly watered flowers. I know that he has picked some of these flowers to grace his dining room table and one small bloom to greet me in the bathroom, a ritual he practices when he expects my visit.

I see him on his stoop, dressed in a blue tank top that matches his eyes and shows off his muscled shoulders. I know he has just showered for me, caressing his body as he washed, thinking of what we would do together.

He is filing his nails in the sunlight as he waits for me. I know what that means: He wants his art- and garden-roughened nails to be smooth for me. We both know that those fingertips will be caressing my most delicate parts and moving inside me to give me pleasure. His studious nail filing has become part of our foreplay, giving me the silent signal that he anticipates our time in bed together and wants to please me. Watching him file his nails, I feel as if he has already been stroking me before we even say hello or smile.

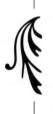

To watch us dance is to hear our hearts speak.
—Hopi Indian saying

My Dancing Man

It took nine months of dancing, walking, and talking before Robert and I became lovers, as you'll read in Chapter 11, "Hunting Ground: In the Dating Game Again (or Still)." Those nine months were foreplay for us, and these activities continue to get us in the mood. We've learned that sex starts before we get home: dancing, exercising together, walking. Physicality is a tremendous turn-on.

Dancing, especially, is sexy—it's vertical eroticism, or, as George Bernard Shaw called it, "a perpendicular expression of a horizontal desire." Dancing is all about celebrating our bodies, expressing ourselves nonverbally, letting our souls soar through our moving bodies. Dancing is also an erotic form of communication with a partner, letting the lift of an arm, the swing of a leg, or the roll of a hip communicate a much more complex and subtle language than words.

When Robert and I dance, whether we're separately line dancing across the room from each other or in a close embrace in a romantic dance, like nightclub two-step, we're aware of our own and each other's body moving expressively, sending each other messages. We entice, seduce, and sometimes just entertain each other with our vertical body language. We're lucky enough to dance together regularly—we teach a line-dance class together, and practice together for fun.

During dry spells between relationships in my past, I would joke with a male friend that dancing was my whole sex life. Indeed, it felt like that: being held in a man's arms, agreeing tacitly to follow wherever and whatever he led (so different from the rest of the way I run my life!), making eye contact—sometimes sensually, sometimes playfully, sometimes just acknowledging the cool dance moves—then saying "thank you" after three minutes and moving on to someone else. Thank goodness for dance!

If dancing isn't a part of your life, I highly recommend it, whether you're partnered, single and looking, or single and satisfied. It adds a dimension of self-expression, body appreciation, and sensuality, whatever your social situation. And it's so much fun! (To find places to dance, search "dance" plus your city or county on the Internet, look at the calendar listings in your newspaper, and find local dance studios, recreation centers, and health clubs in your Yellow Pages.)

Fringe Benefits

"I want to buy you something," Robert tells me. We head for Victoria's Secret, where he picks out a few garments for me to try on. Although no one else in the store looks over twenty-two, no one seems to think it odd that an over-sixty couple is picking out sexy underwear together.

A sales associate unlocks a dressing room for me. "Okay if my sweetie comes in with me?" I ask.

"No, sorry," she says. "He can't go in with you, but you can open the door and show him."

"I didn't understand that," Robert whispers to me.

"She said I can flash you," I explain.

She smiles and nods.

I try on several garments—some silky, some lacy. Not quite right. Then I don a black outfit consisting mostly of fringe.

"Oh, baby!" Robert says when I open the door and shake

Sexually Seasoned Women Speak about How They Get in the Mood

We hug and kiss spontaneously several times a day. That's an easy way to create opportunities to go further. *(Tana, 60)*

He likes to feed me a peeled banana, which I take as much of as I can, as if I were fellating it. *(Joanna, 61)*

I buy new, sexy nightgowns. *(Pepper, 71)*

Nature turns me on. Everything feels warm and beautiful and sexual. The hills of California, all around me beautiful bodies of lovely women, even my photography—a hobby that I took up at fifty-five—reflects my renewal of sexual/sensual awareness. The sounds of birds and animals sound sensual and sexual to me. We went for a walk in a nature preserve, stopping behind a tree and kissing,

my fringe. Decision made. We race for home to take the fringe for a test ride.

Shopping for lingerie together is a great turn-on for us. It's also fun when Robert surprises me with a gift after shopping for me on his own. It stimulates me to know he was thinking of me and how I'd look in the different items he examined. Then we have the fun of trying on the sexy bra or panties or camisole that he chose, and seeing how close his imagination was to the reality of my body.

To make this easy for him, I made sure that our favorite lin-

flirting, walking behind her and telling her she has a beautiful ass. Holding hands. *(Claire, 66)*

When we were first dating and before we had sex, we were kissing and he took my hand, and he put each of my fingers in his mouth, one by one, in a sensual way. I was so turned on by this! *(Melanie, 64)*

I feel sexiest when dancing. *(Ulla, 61)*

We give each other private peeks of our bodies. We'll be fully dressed and discussing something, or eating, or getting ready to part for the day, and one of us will bare a body part quickly (often without stopping the conversation), then cover it again. That sends the other into a tizzy of appreciation. Then we either calm down and go back to what we were doing, or we change course. It's great fun, either way, a little private game we play, and a way to keep affirming that we find each other's body sexy. *(Diana, 62)*

gerie boutique has information about my sizes in its computer, and I also wrote them down for him, at his request, in case he goes to a different store.

Talk to Me

"Do you want me to tell you something sweet?" Robert asks. I nod, and he describes some attribute of mine—a physical or emotional quality, or some way I act in the world—that he finds really special.

Speech [is] the premier sexual lubricant. Humans communicate with each other more often, and over a longer period of time, before they first have consensual sex than any other animal. . . . In short, language evolved primarily because men and women had to negotiate sex.
—Leonard Shlain in *Sex, Time, and Power: How Women's Sexuality Shaped Human Evolution*[1]

The verbal love play that Robert and I enjoy is cozy, intimate, playful, erotic. We have pet names for each other, for our sex toys, and for each other's body parts. We give our own meanings to words, make up words, and devise little bits of ritual wordplay that amuse us and keep us feeling close. Words have such erotic power. Our voices even change when we're talking intimately.

During the first year of our relationship, I was much needier and less secure than I am now. I needed Robert to tell me that he loved me, especially during times of conflict, and Robert resisted this, resenting having to express his love on demand, and frustrated that I always seemed to need more from him. We were in the classic couple's syndrome: fear of abandonment vs. fear of encroachment.

Through much dialogue, a commitment to working things out, and deep love, we melted this hurdle (and others) and grew in beautiful ways, both individually and as a couple. I discovered that I already had what I was asking for, and the less I pushed Robert to tell me that he loved me, the more freely he told me.

Words were the magic key to the kingdom of understanding, and they still remain our most powerful tool. We share problems, thoughts, feelings, fears, and solutions until we've reached resolution. Solving a problem or moving past an obstacle together is not only binding, it's sexy. We often share intense lovemaking afterward. It's word-powered intimacy.

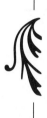

> *For women the best aphrodisiacs are words. The G-spot is in the ears. He who looks for it below there is wasting his time.*
>
> —Isabel Allende

Body Parts in View

From the moment I first met Robert, I was attracted by the curly chest hair I saw peeking out of the V of his shirt. I wanted to stroke it.

Now, whenever I see him in a shirt that exposes some of his chest hair, I have the same yearning to touch him. It takes me back to the long nine months before we became lovers, catching a glimpse of this sexy part of him, the rest hidden from view. The first time we kissed, my hand went straight to that inviting and sexy tuft. It was even softer and more sensual than I had imagined. It's still one of my favorite parts.

When we're dancing together, I'll trail my hand across his chest slowly, making it part of the dance. Sometimes he'll tease me by opening one more top button and letting me see just a little more.

Sexually Seasoned Women Speak about Getting Hot in Public

I swim. Gliding through the water silently is very sexy to me. I especially love a saltwater pool on a ship that's moving through the ocean—I love being rocked in the pool. *(Tina, 61)*

On a recent trip I didn't have the right underwear with me to go with a new dress that I bought. I didn't wear any underwear, and I felt quite sexy. My husband was aroused just knowing that I didn't have any on. I don't believe anyone else was aware. *(Susie, 60)*

Many years ago, we started a fun ritual of always kissing when we find ourselves alone in an elevator. We still do it—and often look up together afterward, to see if perhaps we've been caught on a hidden camera in the elevator. *(Tana, 60)*

I touch other women, straight and lesbian. I hug people and touch their hands. It makes me feel connected and gives me a sensual feeling. *(Claire, 66)*

More Mood-Enhancing Ideas

The first time Robert and I took a weekend trip to a romantic inn, he brought candles to float in the hot tub. When we made love at his house, whether it was morning, afternoon, or nighttime, he lit candles. We had been lovers just a couple of weeks, and I was just learning what a romantic man he is.

Wearing a trim sweater still gets approving looks, and I really enjoy that. My appearance is pretty unremarkable, but I do have nice breasts and get a kick out of having men notice. Being in a conservative business all my working life, I covered up with suits or jackets, and now I don't have to hide my sexuality anymore. *(Mary Ann, 62)*

I can really let myself go when I dance with a good partner, and that makes me feel sexy. My husband doesn't share my love of dancing but is happy when I go dancing with my friends. He knows that I always come home to him a sexier and a happier partner. *(Penny, 60)*

Men call and whistle and wave at me, which turns me on and makes me feel really desirable. Men flirt with me even when they're with another woman; that's cool. *(Catherine, 65)*

When I'm out in public with Eric, I like to imagine him naked. I know his body so well that I can imagine how every body part looks with every move he does. Sometimes I just stare at his nipples, which are very sensitive, and he knows I'm thinking about how he responds when I pinch them. He's much more subtle—I can't tell he's staring at my breasts or hips until he tells me later. *(Diana, 62)*

I think women are biologically programmed to find romance sexy. Remember even back in high school, when words of love (especially written in a note!), a corsage, or an unexpected gift made our hearts flutter? Now that we're older and we need more warming up, romance goes a long way towards heating up the bedroom. Here are some more romantic pathways to try:

• Make sex dates for the best time of day for you, whether it's the late morning, midafternoon, or nighttime, whenever you're most lively.

• Massage each other's feet slowly.

• Make a tape or CD of romantic music from the era of your youth. Dance to it, or play it in the background when you make love.

• Make a tape or CD of popular music from your youth, romantic or not. Dance to it, giggle to it, or just plain have fun feeling young to it.

• Take a bath together, or caress each other when one of you is in the bath and the other isn't.

• Accessorize: Use candles, mirrors, flowers, or silk to set a sexy and romantic mood.

• Choose a special greeting card for no occasion at all, except that you're in love (or lust), and write a special message on it.

• Shop for sex toys together.

• Take a romantic dance class together, such as tango or nightclub two-step, and practice frequently.

• Leave a love message on your lover's answering machine when you know he or she isn't home.

• Wear sexy lingerie under ordinary clothes, and flash your lover a preview.

• Touch your lover's back softly for a very long time.

• Listen. Be your lover's best friend.

Public Sex—for Real

You probably flipped to this chapter titled "Public Sex Acts" thinking it would contain stories about women actually having sex out in public, perhaps with other people watching. If you've read this far, you deserve such stories, so here are a couple from my interviewees who enjoy one form of public sex—group sex parties:

I go to parties at a swing house. The house is very comfortable—like being in someone's home, except for the containers of condoms. This party scene is a mix, age-wise, most in the middle-age range. I am one of the older ones. I met Charlie, my current partner, there. I spent most of the evening with him, and I still get those rushes down my spine whenever I think about him. Now that I've met Charlie, I don't really care if I party with other men as long as I get my time with him. But I will party, just to see what's out there. So far, other partners just don't have the finesse that he does. Our agreement is that we will do what—or whom—we want. When I was younger, I never thought that I could share my partner with others, but now I think monogamy is not realistic. We haven't had many in-depth conversations yet. Mine consists of "Oh my god," repeated at length. (Kaycee, 66)

I like to go to sex parties. At these events, we all agree to practice safe sex, even those couples who are "fluid-bonded"—those who have been tested for STDs and don't use condoms or other barriers at home. Typically a group of sixty to eighty people will attend—hetero, gay male, lesbian, and those of any orientation who are into light S&M. So there's a lot of variety in what goes on. The parties happen in a big, open room, with exhibitionistic people being watched by those who enjoy watching. I enjoy both. At a sex party once, I got on my hands and knees and told a woman friend to get a couple of men to have sex with me. I didn't want to see them or know who they were. She started with a dildo in a harness. Then, after the men started, I didn't like it and asked them to stop. It was a good fantasy, though, and it's still a fantasy I enjoy. (Laura, 63)

Claire, Sixty-six, and Her Ocean Lover

The ocean was roaring and sending huge sprays against the craggy rocks where we sat, holding each other. We could feel the force of the ocean coming at us. We were turned on by the foam licking the rocks and the waves coming in different colors around us. I whispered, "Why not?" I unbuttoned my jeans, and she reached inside to the warmth and wetness that awaited her hand. She began to massage me as the ocean was massaging the rocks, appearing to soften them into puddles of clay. As my body rose to welcome her hand, I came into my pleasure with her breathing softly into my ear. My hand grasped a handful of sand, feeling its wetness and warmth. I felt that I had become part of the beautiful scene with the sounds of the roaring ocean and the soft sunlight on our bodies. It was as if I had the ocean all to myself, softly caressing me with all her magnificent power. The ocean was my most awesome lover on this sensual day.

CHAPTER 8

Beds Afire: Stoking the Slower-Burning Flame

All moderation should be thrown aside, the act should be prolonged for as long as possible, and to make the fires of desire burn even more brightly, all manner of caresses, cries, and other stimulants to love should be used.

—Kama Sutra

I rub moisturizing lotion gently into Robert's skin. I love seeing him standing naked before me, body clean and warm from his shower. I want to taste all of it. He stands open to me, arms relaxed at his sides or raised for me when I lift them. His legs are apart to give me access to thighs, calves, buttocks. I sense him trusting and vulnerable. This is incredibly sexy to me. We are so quiet that I can listen to his breath.

I like to stand in the sunlight from a window when he "moisturizes" me, as we call it in our sweet, private language of love. The cold lotion on my warm skin is shocking in a wonderfully sensual way. His hands glide slowly over my body, piece by piece, his eyes on the section of skin he is touching. "I know every part of you," he says. This turns me on—he knows my body, every inch, and he loves and desires me. Life doesn't get any better than that.

I love it when we shower together and he washes my hair. I feel childlike, my head in his hands, his strong fingers working the shampoo into lather. Later he washes my feet as I lift my toes to give him access.

These ministrations are so special and sexy that we are careful not to let them become routine. We keep them for languid, lengthy mornings or afternoons when we have decided to set aside work and give each other full attention.

Slow Burn

We've learned how to slow down sex, make it sensual and languorous as well as hot and passionate. I used to feel needy, urgent, and, frankly, self-centered. Now I feel more relaxed about sex—more giving and more open.

I've learned to practice slow sex out of necessity—my arousal time is much slower than it used to be. I need much more warm-up time, more touching all over before we get to my hot spots. Sometimes it feels like the sensation recedes out of reach, like watching ocean waves in the distance through a smudged window. I remember what it feels like, but the sensation is blurred, muffled. In my thirties, I'd jump out of my skin at the hot fire of an intimate touch. Now it's a slow, sensuous warmth, gradually spreading. Sex feels less localized, more whole body.

When my relationship with Robert first became sexual, I was embarrassed at how long I took to get aroused and how much longer after that it took to bring me to orgasm. After one lengthy session, I apologized that I had taken so long. Silly me, I thought he must have been bored. He looked at me with that *Are you out of your mind?* look and said, "I don't care if it takes three weeks, as long as I can take breaks sometimes to change positions and get something to eat."

Lube Power

I used to be embarrassed that I no longer lubricated and had to resort (as I saw it) to using a lubricant in addition to wearing an estrogen ring. Robert helped me change my attitude by making the lubricant part of love play. He applies it with caresses to me and to himself, enjoying the sensuality of fingers gliding over slippery skin. It is a turn-on for us both, and a great source of pleasure.

Lubricants—if you haven't tried them—are slippery lotions designed for sexual enhancement and comfort that give you back the moist slickness that hormonal depletion may have taken away. We've tried many different kinds, sampling them from Blowfish (www.blowfish.com) and from local woman-friendly sex shops (see the Resources section in the Appendix). Don't restrict yourself to the few choices at your local drugstore—there are dozens of options that vary in slipperiness, staying power, feel, and heaviness. (I'm told they also vary in taste, but we prefer to apply lubricant *after* oral sex.) Our personal preference is Liquid Silk, though yours might be different. Let me know if you have a favorite (email me at joan@joanprice.com), and I'll include an annotated list in a future book.

Intimate Interior Design

No, I'm not suggesting that you redecorate your vaginal walls. Rather, put special sexual aids, such as your vibrator and lube, in elegant containers.

I have a lovely woven basket for our lubricants, for example. Every glimpse of the basket on my nightstand makes me think about the last time we opened it—and anticipate the next time.

I wear an estrogen ring internally. Although instructions say that the ring doesn't have to be removed during intercourse, Robert feels it, so I remove it before we have sex. I used to store the ring in a plastic deli tub—how unsexy!—until Robert presented me with a special estrogen-ring box. On it he had painted an open flower, with what looks like an erect clitoris in its center (or so I see it!) and a heart on the bottom.

Holiday Festivities

Robert and I celebrated Valentine's Day 2005 by staying in bed—making love, holding each other, napping, reading to each other, making love again—all day, just getting up for pee breaks and snacks. By midafternoon, we were starved. I warmed up the dinner Robert had prepared the day before. Then we

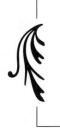

It is not sex that gives the pleasure but the lover.
—Marge Piercy, novelist, essayist, and poet

went back to bed until midevening, when we rose to eat again and to watch *American Idol*.

Kiss Me Forever

I remember the long, frenzied kissing sessions of my younger days, when the right technique (although that seems too crass a term to describe kissing) would stir electric sparks through my body.

Now I have the best kissing sessions of my life, yet my depleted hormones don't send those same sparks. It's a different experience—as emotional and spiritual as physical. Extended kissing sends me into a lulled zone where Robert and I are totally one.

Maybe it's oxytocin, the feel-good hormone and bonding chemical. Oxytocin peaks during orgasm and is responsible for that euphoric feeling you get when you cuddle afterward. My oxytocin seems to surge during kissing, too. When we kiss and

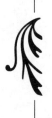

A kiss is a lovely trick designed by nature to stop speech when words become superfluous.
—Ingrid Bergman

Sexually Seasoned Women Describe What Turns Them On

I've learned to enjoy being aroused for a considerable time without needing to jump into bed immediately. We often tease each other for a day or two before a scheduled get-together. I like a gentle and loving approach to sex, with much caressing and teasing. Later on, I like oral sex. He's never in a hurry, which is great. *(Mary Ann, 62)*

I love being stroked. I love a man who does everything slowly and gently and kisses for a long time, teasing me, indirectly arousing me, and not hitting my most erogenous zones immediately. I go into an altered state. *(Erica, 62)*

Sometimes Eric surprises me with a striptease. He puts together a costume (easily shed) and performs a sensuous dance for me, removing or opening clothing to show off his most attractive attributes but not letting me touch. When at last he sheds the last bit of clothing and welcomes my touch, I am ravenous for him. *(Diana, 62)*

I really like my toes sucked. He has a bit of a foot fetish, so we're well matched. I like to be tied up and blindfolded and just be his because I trust him so implicitly. I'm such a strong woman out in the world that it's nice to give myself to him and not have to be in charge. *(Monica, 60)*

It really turns me on when my lover just turns down the covers and looks at me. He spreads my legs and looks closely at my vagina, then slowly begins to touch it. *(Penny, 60)*

I almost always have an orgasm with whole-body massages. One time in particular was a turn-on because most of the massage was concentrated on my legs and buttocks, and when it moved up to my neck and shoulders, I experienced an amazing orgasm. *(Ulla, 61)*

The best enhancer for me is a little pot a half hour beforehand. I don't really feel sexy unless I'm high. I've tried medication, which didn't work. When I spoke to my doctor, she said if pot works, stick with pot. *(Pepper, 71)*

I like foreplay. My clitoris is my sexual thermometer. If it's not stimulated a lot, nothing happens. I could forego intercourse and just play slap-and-tickle and be happy. *(Catherine, 65)*

Touching. Feeling. Fingers and tongue. Never anything abrupt. Good timing. Our inventiveness never pales, our joyous couplings never become commonplace. *(Rachel, 62)*

Turning him on turns me on! My partner is a strong-willed, take-charge person in life, and sometimes he likes to be submissive in sex. On special occasions, I put his wrists and ankles in soft restraints and tie them to the bedposts. Then I can do whatever I want to him as he lies there, spread-eagled, his gorgeous body on display for my pleasure. I can stroke him lightly and flutter my tongue over any part of him. *(Kassie, 62)*

continued on next page

continued from page 117

I have always been a woman who wants to have sex out in nature. I have had sex on the farthest rock sticking out into the ocean. When the stags rut in Armstrong Woods in Guerneville, California, it is a great place to have sex— after they are gone, of course—because you can feel the sexual energy there. The sand dunes at Bodega Headlands, also in California—that's another good place. I plan to take K to many of these places. It's risky, of course, but having been a lesbian since age twelve, I know how to take risks—I wasn't supposed to have sex with other women, remember. *(Claire, 66)*

He's a pretty dominant partner, and he holds me down a lot. When he sees a loose hand floating around, he grabs my wrist and holds onto it. I like that a lot. I'm not a submissive person, but it turns me on to be restrained. If we had some soft ropes and things, we'd use them, but we've never gotten around to getting them. It gets him hard to spank me, and it turns me on. He knows just where to swat, the sweet spot, just above the crease between cheek and thigh. *(Nina, 67)*

He lets me know every day in every way that he loves me. *(Joanna, 61)*

kiss, I feel bonding and love washing over me, enveloping me like a warm bath of sensuality, and there's nothing I'd rather be doing than kissing the man I love.

In my youth, kissing was frenzied, and it had a goal: to ignite me to the next step. Now, though I do love the next step (and every step), I could also be content just kissing.

Games in the Dark

Robert and I have a kissing game we play in the dark. After turning off the lights, and before our eyes adjust to the dark, we say, "Let's kiss." Then we each aim our mouth at where we think the other person's mouth must be. We're so in love, so connected, that obviously our internal sensors can find the other's mouth, right? Wrong—we invariably miss, connecting mouth to ear or chin or empty air, and we sputter into gales of laughter. We try again and again until our mouths join and we feel peaceful and bonded.

Laughter is not only sexy, sometimes it is sex: connection on a deep level. We have a number of games we play that have evolved out of our love of laughter.

Lips Off Limits

March 27, 2005. Robert and I haven't been able to kiss for a week because my lip broke out in a herpes sore. Robert has reached age sixty-eight without either oral or genital herpes, and I'm doing my best to keep it that way by keeping my lip—which breaks out every year or so—away from him. I started protecting him when I felt that first tingle, before any visible signs. Sometimes it goes away and doesn't break open at that point, but I never take any chances. This time, it erupted into a

My Brain Chemicals Made Me Do It

According to anthropologist/evolutionary biologist/love specialist Helen Fisher, PhD, different brain chemicals dominate different stages of love:

1. Lust (craving sexual gratification) is driven by androgens and estrogens.

2. Attraction (romantic or passionate love, euphoria, intense craving for loved one) is driven by high dopamine and norepinephrine levels and low serotonin.

3. Attachment (calm, connection, stability) is driven by the hormones oxytocin and vasopressin.

High levels of oxytocin and vasopressin may interfere with dopamine and norepinephrine pathways, Dr. Fisher explains, which may explain why attachment grows as mad passion fades. It makes sense to me that when our androgen and estrogen levels recede with age, we're more in touch with the "attachment" stage.

I contacted Dr. Fisher and asked her about the association of oxytocin and kissing. She replied:

big, ugly lesion with yellow goop, and I was glad I had kept my lips away from his mucus membranes.

It was tough, though. Yesterday we made love without kissing, but we were kissing with our minds. "I'm pretending I'm kissing you," I told him. "I'm pretending I'm kissing you, too," he said.

Saturday Night

Robert and I dance a lot during the week—he comes to my line dance classes, and often we learn a new dance or practice

I don't know if levels of oxytocin rise with kissing; I don't think anyone does. I would think they would rise if you were in a long-term attachment. But if you are in the throes of intense romantic passion with someone new, levels of dopamine and norepinephrine may rise instead. I would say that kissing is "situational"—the hormones and neurotransmitters involved will vary depending on the state of the relationship. We do know that orgasm increases levels of oxytocin in women. And this probably contributes to the feeling of union and attachment after orgasm with a partner one loves.

Dr. Fisher is also the author of four books on the biology of love. These books don't deal specifically with older women, but are fascinating nonetheless. You can check them out at her website, www.helenfisher.com. Meanwhile, you can blame it on brain chemicals if you want, but these drugs are legal—so enjoy them!

together at other times. Our favorite Saturday evening activity is very different: we listen to the radio together.

Specifically, we snuggle together naked and listen to National Public Radio's *Selected Shorts*, readings of classic and modern short stories. Both the readers and the stories are terrific, and it's a wonderful way to be quiet together, winding down and sharing an experience while feeling the touch and heat of each other's bodies. I confess that I sometimes fall asleep before the story ends, not due to fatigue but because

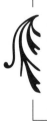

> *Ancient lovers believed a kiss would literally unite their souls because the spirit was said to be carried in one's breath.*
>
> —Eve Glicksman

I feel so peaceful snuggling with my lover and listening to a bedtime story.

Claire Keeps Her Long-Distance Relationship Sizzling

Claire, sixty-six, is about to relocate to be with the woman she loves, whom she met via the Internet. Until they can be together, here's how they keep the fires burning:

> *We write explicit emails, hot and heavy. I love to write, so I write her a love letter every morning. We give each other lots of love and sexual energy in our emails. I have so much inside of me that hasn't been expressed, and I want to express it all. I'm making up for lost time.*
>
> *On our last trip together, we bought candles, and we burn them when we're instant messaging. It makes us feel connected. We IM every day and call at least once a week.*
>
> *We get the same movie—preferably one that is sensuous and fun—and watch it at the same time and then talk about it the next day. We are both reading the same poets— May Sarton, Mary Oliver, Adrienne Rich—and we discuss them when we IM or talk on the phone. We both have each*

Our Secret Sex Lives: Sexually Seasoned Women Describe Their Erotic Fantasies

I fantasize about being dominated. In real life, I'd scream bloody murder, file lawsuits, shoot the prick. In fantasy, it's very powerful. I love having my wrists held down. In reality, I take no shit. *(Rachel, 62)*

I want us to make love on a secluded beach in the Caribbean for a really long time, be naked all the time, put flowers all over each other, and lick rum off of each other's thighs. *(Monica, 60)*

I'm making love with a group of men. They're all fascinated and excited by me and want nothing more than to pleasure me. They're all in it to please me—the younger men want to discover what pleases a woman; the older ones want to show that they already know. This fantasy turns me on, but I wouldn't want to really experience it. I've tried a threesome, and it wasn't nearly as much fun as my fantasy. *(Lexie, 63)*

I fantasize about being tied to a tree and having several men fondle me one at a time while the others watch, bringing me to orgasm over and over. *(Ulla, 61)*

other's pictures near our beds and always say goodnight to each other through the pictures.

I have great fantasies during the day. I fantasize about her when we can't be together. I imagine making love in the vineyard amongst things that are growing, the sensual feeling of the sun on my body. I've sent her a tape of me masturbating.

We praise each other for our patience and courage to do this at all. We are each other's heroines.

Try to incorporate some sexual fantasies into your lovemaking. So if you have always wanted to do it in a rocking chair or on a blanket in front of the fireplace, or you want to play strip poker, cover your partner in whipping cream, or give a gentle spanking, why not try it?
—Sue Johanson in *Sex, Sex, and More Sex*[1]

Extended Foreplay

Robert and I live in separate houses five minutes apart. I wonder if we would feel as sexy about each other if we lived together. Although it's sometimes frustrating not to be able to kiss or hold him each night when I go to sleep and each morning when I wake, I find our times together to be that much more exciting because they don't happen automatically.

We've discovered that sex works best when we schedule it,

make time for it, clear away our busy calendars for it. We turn off our computers and phone ringers. We make dates, anticipate our times together, plan for them, fantasize about them, and tantalize each other by phone by murmuring about what we'd like to do. What we give up in spontaneity, we make up for with constant mental foreplay!

Part of our foreplay ostensibly has nothing to do with sex. We delight in doing things for each other, giving each other little presents and pleasures. He phones me one morning to say, "I cooked last night and made enough for you. I can bring it by on the way to my studio." I am moved and happy that he cooked for two, even though we weren't together, and love being surprised with today's dinner—organic vegetables (lots of mushrooms), noodles, tofu, and freshly grated ginger.

When I grocery shop, I always buy a few items that I know Robert likes—biscotti from our local Wildflour bakery, Trader Joe's trail mix, or Peet's coffee beans. I tuck them in a bag to give to him the next time I see him. We have special bags that we keep trading back and forth with little treats for each other.

He takes a shipment to the post office for me. I address his art-show postcards. I buy a book for him that I think he'll like and blue shirts that match his eyes. He buys me lingerie, earrings, and necklaces. I buy him fishnet bikini underwear from The Sensuality Shoppe, the local sensual boutique (see Appendix).

I have never felt so unselfish, not only in sex but also in the whole gestalt of our relationship. I get great pleasure doing some little thing that will elicit a smile, or save him time, or take a task off his mind.

We deliberately make each other laugh, and hilarity is one

of our favorite ways to come together. We've developed a lovers' language: words and phrases that have special meanings for us, or elicit memories, or just make us laugh. We've learned to listen between the words.

We dance with our bodies, our words, and our vulnerabilities, and we seek out opportunities to please each other. All of this is foreplay.

When we finally come together for sex, it's as if we've been making love for days.

Encarta Dictionary defines "foreplay" as "Mutual sexual stimulation that takes place before intercourse."[2] It's funny that there's no word for "sexual stimulation that takes place for days before intercourse" or for "sexual stimulation that takes place whether intercourse does or not."

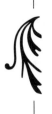

Sex is hardly ever just about sex.
—Shirley MacLaine

CHAPTER 9

Plug In, Turn On:

The Quick Version of Everything You Need to Know about Sex Toys

Power Up

What do I love about vibrators?

- They're great.
- They intensify sensations.
- They increase the probability of orgasm.
- They increase the intensity of orgasm.

• They're great (did I say that?) for couple sex as well as solitary sex.

Emotionally, I love sex as much as I ever have. Physically, my hormone depletion has subdued my sexual sensations and made them more difficult to access. The best solution for me is a loving relationship, lots and lots of kissing and touching, and the help of a well-chosen, well-placed vibrator.

In my younger days, I used a vibrator for solo sex but never with a partner. I would have been too embarrassed, and besides, guys were nervous about vibrators. They thought we were trying to replace them with machinery that could go harder, stronger, and longer than they could. For me, that was (and is) unrelated to the attraction of vibrators. Rather, it's the deep, electrifying sensation that reverberates through my body and brings my nerve endings to life so that my physical high matches the emotional one.

A Short History of Vibrators

From the time of Hippocrates until the turn of the twentieth century, physicians believed that women suffered from the disease "hysteria" (a word that comes from the Greek, meaning "suffering uterus"). This affliction involved emotional distress and irritability due to "pelvic heaviness" (sexual frustration). To treat this disease during Victorian times, doctors performed genital massage until the patient experienced "hysterical paroxysm" (orgasm).

In the late nineteenth century, the first vibrators appeared and were sold to doctors (after all, hands-on hysteria treatment took far too much time). Vibrators were later advertised to women for self-treatment of hysteria and, by 1920, for health, vigor, youth, beauty, and a variety of health conditions from headaches to tuberculosis.

After vibrators started appearing in "blue movies" in the 1920s, showing women pleasuring themselves, their cover was blown, and mass-market advertising stopped for a few decades. Vibrators reappeared disguised as personal-care appliances for self-massage (you know, for a sore calf muscle or more vibrant skin), with pictures of women massaging their cheeks for a rosy glow. Dildos were clearly for sex, but vibrators hummed away, respectably camouflaged.

I visit the Museum of Sex in New York (www.museumofsex .com) and view a display of vibrators from 1900 to 1920, including a "blood circulator" that resembles a manual eggbeater without the beaters. You had to be really determined (or very quick!) to keep that thing going long enough to achieve your goal, and I can imagine the carpal-tunnel syndrome that resolved users developed! Fast-forward to modern inventions: The museum displays prototypes of penetrating sex machines that the user would mount or lie back and "receive," with names like Monkey Rocker and Thrillhammer.

Toys Are Us: My Personal Vibrator History

I bought my first vibrator in my thirties at Macy's: a "personal care" product for, uh, "massage." The instructions said nothing about using it for sex, but, wink-wink, I knew.

For decades, I collected vibrators, trying to find *the* model that would do it for me. I don't remember if I started with the Wahl (which I named Wally), with its many intriguing attachments, or the Hitachi Magic Wand (named Big Buzzy), but after buying the first one, I quickly bought another.

Over the next few years, I filled three nightstand drawers with vibrators of all sorts, both plug-in and battery-operated. I had vibrators in the shape of a penis, egg, wand, rabbit, and probably more I'm forgetting. I must have tried every type of vibrator on the planet, not because I love variety but because it was difficult to find *the* one for me. I've always preferred the strength of plug-in rather than battery-operated sex toys, and now that I'm older, I need the most intensity possible from my toys. A "light touch" is pleasant, but if my goal is orgasm, it's got to be strong.

A few years ago, I cleaned out my drawers, threw out the thirty-year-old attachments that had deteriorated into flakes of plastic, discarded the toys I didn't really like, and kept only my favorites. I hated to throw this large collection in the trash, but I figured neither Goodwill nor my local consignment store would accept used sex toys, and they weren't old enough to donate to Good Vibrations's antique vibrator museum (www.goodvibes.com).

I decided I didn't need all these extra toys anymore because I've discovered my favorite: the Eroscillator (www.eroscillator .com), an oscillating plug-in designed for clitoral stimulation. It feels great—intense and focused, with its smooth, rotating motion—and it is easy to hold, easy to aim, and easy to adjust intensity during the act. A twelve-foot-long cord makes it work in hotel rooms, where the outlet might be half a wall away. Best of all, the long, slim handle and small vibrating part make it simple and comfortable to use with a partner. It's expensive—$120 to almost $200, depending on attachments—but worth every penny.

Because the Eroscillator is endorsed by Dr. Ruth Westheimer and her picture is on the box, I named mine "Dr. Ruth."

Electrifying Sex: Using Sex Toys with a Partner

At some point after Robert and I became sexual, I asked if he'd be open to using a vibrator with me. His response was a definitive, absolute, "No! I don't want a machine in the middle of our lovemaking!" He had had no experience with what he called "appliances," and they didn't fit with his feelings about lovemaking as natural and spiritual. When I showed him my vibrator, it seemed like a noisy, mechanical thing.

Robert would make me come with his fingers before or after intercourse—I couldn't come during intercourse at all. My sensations just weren't strong enough anymore to bring me over the top unless I had really strong, direct, and focused clitoral stimulation. He kept asking if there was anything he could do during intercourse so that I could come that way, and my answer was always, "Only if we use a vibrator at the same time."

Finally, he agreed to try it. The ease of giving me an orgasm and the intensity of my pleasure won him over. We've used it ever since, and it's part of our love play. Now Robert will say in the middle of sex, "Let's get my buddy, Dr. Ruth!"

We make our preparation part of sex play. Robert takes the vibrator out of the drawer, plugs it in, and turns it on, running it over his own skin. Then it stays on the nightstand in plain sight, easy for either of us to reach.

Your First Vibrator:
The Possibilities of Pleasure

By Carol Queen, PhD

Vibrator shopping could be called the mechanical equivalent of choosing a lover. There's no one best vibrator. If you're not sure what you like, try two different types to start to figure out your erotic priorities. Share your preferences with the staff of a woman-friendly sex shop—they have expertise and can offer helpful guidance.

There are plug-in electric vibrators, also called massagers, and battery-operated vibes. The plug-in ones are bigger, heavier, stronger, and usually louder than battery models. Many women love the Hitachi Magic Wand because of its vibration strength and large-size head, which diffuses the vibrations over a larger area, though some find it just too big and overwhelming.

The plug-ins may be motor-operated wands or small, cake-mixer-shaped coil vibrators. The coils are smaller, milder, and quieter than the wands, but they also have a smaller head (the part that you place against the part you want to vibrate). This concentrates the vibrations into a small area, so some folks find the coils feel even stronger than the wands. Imagine the difference between touching the clitoris with one finger and placing a whole palm over the vulva. The difference is sort of like that—only, of course, vibrational. Electric vibes are appliance quality and will last a long time.

Battery vibes offer an embarrassment of riches—there are about thirteen jillion kinds. At some stores, such as Good Vibrations, you can turn the vibes on and feel their vibration. You might like your vibration strong, mild, or medium.

Do you want one for penetration? Some battery vibes are designed for external stimulation only, like the Japanese-made Pocket Rocket styles, while others can be used in the vagina or anus. Vaginal vibration is not as powerful for most women as clitoral, so if you like the feeling of penetration, you might be happy with a dildo. Twice as Nice, a style that bridges the gap, has a clitoral vibe (usually molded in the shape of an animal) and a shaft. The two simultaneous sources of stimulation are heaven for a lot of women.

If you want penetration, do you want the vibrator to be soft or hard? You can choose from nearly realistic, penis-like textures to hard plastic or Lucite. Some look penis-y, while others are shaped like rockets or more fanciful forms: octopi, mermaids, wiener dogs, and other wacky styles.

The bullet-style vibrator—shaped like an egg or a small, soft-edged cylinder—is made of hard plastic, which usually has a strong buzz. The bullets feel pretty intense, the smallest ones even more than the larger ones, with less diffusion and more focus. These are usually powered by a battery pack attached with a cord. These vibes can be worn in special underwear or pouches, or simply held over the area you want buzzed. They're small enough to fit between two people easily. (You can use any vibe this way, but the bigger ones require positioning accordingly—the Hitachi is a foot long!) Do you want it waterproof? What color or pattern? Smooth or textured? Straight or G-spot curvy? Small or large? Fast, buzzy vibe, or slow? Trying them out is fun—they're toys! Soon enough, you'll find one you'll love.[1]

Carol Queen, PhD (www.carolqueen.com), is a writer, speaker, educator, and activist with a doctorate degree in sexology.

Robert Speaks: Making the Love Bed

I read this chapter aloud to Robert, and acknowledge the tremendous change he has made in accepting sex toys in our lovemaking. "What is it like for you?" I ask. He responds:

I tease that our sex toys are "appliances," but I really think of them as attributes of lovemaking. When you're in the bathroom getting ready, I do what I think of as "making the love bed": I prepare the accessories we use. I take the protective cover off the wedge pillow, and I get out the lubricant. I plug in Dr. Ruth and run the vibrator over my own skin so you hear the noise and know what's coming. I like to feel it myself, too. It's a sign of my readiness to make love to you.

I see all this as preparing for receiving you. The making of the love nest may not involve lace coverlets or strewn rose petals but rather vibrators, lubricants, and special pillows designed to save the back. Still, the thought is the same.

Eros Therapy

I don't like the term "feminine sexual dysfunction"—who said we're all supposed to function in any specific way? But I was intrigued by the idea of a device called Eros Therapy (www.nugyn.com), a gentle vacuum that is FDA-approved for treating FSD by improving sensitivity and sexual response and satisfaction. This device is not a vibrator or a sex toy, the literature insists, but a mechanism that increases blood flow to the clitoris and external genitalia. It's available by prescription only, and it costs $400. What device could be worth that much? I wondered.

Robert always responds with reservation and trepidation to any device that he worries may impede the natural sexual development of our lovemaking. When he first saw the Eros Therapy device, he said, "It looks so clinical. Couldn't they make it look more attractive, like a flower or something?" Okay, it doesn't look like a flower. It looks a little like a plastic, palm-size bar of Dove soap. You attach a clear, miniature cup, described very well in a magazine as a doll-size oxygen mask. Robert thinks it looks like a miniature feed bag attached to an oversize computer mouse.

I had assumed it could be used during sex, but the instructions said one minute on, one minute off, five times in a row, either as a solitary activity or prior to intercourse. I tried it on my own at first, while Robert read the newspaper beside me in bed, every so often casting his eyes my way to see if I was doing anything interesting. I wasn't—just pressing the cup over my clitoris and experimenting with placement and amount of suction, and sometimes uttering, "Oh!" It was a pleasant sensation to have my clitoris sucked by a vacuum device, but it didn't bring me to uncontrolled fits of ecstasy.

The next morning, we prepared to make love—choosing our lube, positioning our wedge pillow and Dr. Ruth within reach, and showering and shaving, each activity a slow, sexy part of foreplay. I decided to see if another round of Eros Therapy might pay off in—what? Increased sensation? Natural lubrication? Faster orgasm? I wasn't sure what to expect as I pumped blood into my sweet spot.

"Whoa, you've grown!" said Robert, observing my clitoral engorgement. As he touched me, wow, I did indeed have increased sensation. In fact, I felt the youthful zinging and tingling that had become so rare in my hormone-deprived sex organs. I loved the feeling!

Sexually Seasoned Women Speak about Using Sex Toys

Amazing Grace is the name of my vibrator, which I've had for over twenty-two years. The name came to me one night when I felt so relieved of stress and realized what a comfort it was to me. It's just one of those cheap massagers with various attachments. I tried all the attachments, but they weren't very satisfying. So, one day I tried using the half-inch piece of steel without the attachments. It has a very low but steady vibration, and the best part is that it gets warmer and warmer with use. By the time I have a climax, it is as hot as it would feel if someone else were stimulating me, doing what I told her I wanted. Amazing Grace has helped me to know myself in a very important way. Because I know what feels good to me, I can allow another woman to know how to pleasure me. Of course, the reason it works so well is that I can control the use of it. I have been with women who thought they knew what I needed instead of listening to what I was telling them I wanted. *(Claire, 66)*

My vibrator's name is Mr. Buzzy. My partner named it. *(Phoebe, 64)*

I have a large vibrator with hard rubber pieces that fit on it. They are different shapes—curved and so on. I don't have much feeling on the inside at all, it's all in the clitoris. *(Melanie, 64)*

At first Eric resisted using a vibrator with me, but after he saw how powerful my orgasm was, he was as thrilled as I was. Now he reaches for it, stimulates his own nipples and mine, and then places it where I like it. At a certain point, I take over holding the vibrator so I can adjust the pressure, placement, and speed so it's just right. Sometimes we have simultaneous orgasms during intercourse, an impossibility without the vibrator. It's wonderful—I have a strong, screaming orgasm, and in the middle of it he starts to come, his song joining mine. *(Diana, 62)*

Hitachi Magic Wand is great for orgasms. So is my bidet. I learned about massaging the G-spot at a Tantric yoga seminar about eight years ago, and I find that that is another way to get a release. I've tried dildos but haven't found them very helpful. *(Phoebe, 64)*

I tend to masturbate more when I have a regular partner. The more orgasms I'm having, the more I want to have. It's not unusual for me to masturbate away and have one more for the road when he's in the bathroom throwing away the condom. *(Nina, 67)*

When my husband is traveling on business, I sometimes use the vibrator to help me go to sleep. It's more like a sleeping pill than a satisfying sexual experience. *(Susie, 60)*

We haven't used any sex toys recently, but we have used some in the past, like a dildo and a cucumber. We had a vibrator when we were younger, but we lost it! *(Penny, 60)*

Sexually Seasoned Women Speak about Buying and Using Sex Toys

I love Blowfish (www.blowfish.com) and read their mailings avidly. I've never walked into a sex shop. *(Rachel, 62)*

Good Vibrations is a short distance from my home, and the people there are so great. I never thought that I would walk into a store and ask for condoms for blowjobs. *(Kaycee, 66)*

I use my hands. I don't have any sex toys. I've been curious. Years ago, I went into a sex store and laughed, but I never bought anything. *(Matilda, 78)*

Eric and I went together to Good Vibrations in San Francisco. We couldn't believe the variety of dildo shapes, colors, and sizes, and the domination contraptions that we had never seen before. A young man with piercings asked if he could help us. Eric asked about anal toys, which he'd

Although I can't say that my orgasm came any faster (and who cares about that when you're having fun?), it was stronger, and the path there was filled with plenty of rushes of strong sensation. I continue to use Eros before sex, and my orgasms are definitely stronger.

Worth the money? To me, absolutely. Of course, consult your own physician to see whether Eros Therapy is appropriate for you, and since we're all different, your mileage may vary.

never used before. The young man showed us to a wall display of sex toys for anal insertion and described the attributes of several, letting Eric handle them. He was explicit and at the same time respectful and professional. If a man the age of his grandfather asking about butt plugs fazed the young guy, he didn't show it. Eric bought a toy he named "Purple Penis." *(Diana, 62)*

I once went with my partner to a men's sex shop but felt strange. Then a women's sex shop, called A Woman's Touch, opened in Madison, Wisconsin. Both my partner and I have been in it together and separately. It's comfortable to be in, and it has scents, feathers, sexy nightgowns, and all kinds of sex-enhancing things that appeal to women. *(Pepper, 71)*

I am not entirely comfortable going in shops, but I will work on it. *(Claire, 66)*

Now that I'm single, I am very, very tempted to get a dildo—not a vibrator; the noise would annoy me. *(Rachel, 62)*

Woman-Friendly Sex Shops

"We don't call this a 'sex shop,'" Gina Williams, cofounder of The Sensuality Shoppe in Sebastopol, California, tells me. "We're an 'erotic boutique.'" I learn that a county ordinance specifies that a "sex shop" must sell fifty percent or more "adult material." Since The Sensuality Shoppe is filled with lingerie, body-care products, books, and jewelry as well as sex toys, it can't—and doesn't want to—call itself a "sex shop."

Four Tips for Toys:
A Guide for Women of a Certain Age
By Ellen Barnard, MSSW

1. As we grow older, it becomes harder to get blood into the clitoris. Vibrators are excellent for helping you get aroused faster and for helping you have orgasms when it's hard to have them through oral or manual stimulation alone. For women with diminished sensation, one of the newer "gyrating" styles brings a lot of blood into the clitoris. If you're on a medication in the Prozac family or blood pressure medication, you'll want a vibrator that is on the strong end: a plug-in-the-wall style or a very strong, battery-operated one. (One psychiatrist I know said that vibrators should be handed out along with antidepressants—they make the difference between having orgasms and not having them when you're on these drugs.)

2. Dildos are good for your health. Regardless of your age, it is good for your vagina to get regular massage through penetration. Once you're past menopause, the vaginal skin thins more quickly, and a good session with a dildo once or

I'll continue to use the term "woman-friendly sex shop" to refer to both neighborhood and online retail establishments that sell sex toys, among other sexual enhancements, and make women feel comfortable shopping there. If you're looking in your own Yellow Pages, be creative in your word choices if what you find under "sex shop" looks too sleazy for your comfort. Check out your alternative weekly newspaper. Ask other women. The stores you're looking for are out there.

twice a week will help you maintain your vaginal skin and its flexibility. Choose one that is about as wide as the number of fingers that you can insert comfortably into your vagina when aroused. Silicone dildos are the easiest to clean.

3. Add good moisturizing lubricant to every toy you put inside you to protect your skin from damage and increase the sensitivity of your nerve endings. Avoid glycerin if you get yeast infections, and use a silicone-based lubricant only with toys not made with silicone. Don't use oil; it's not good for your vagina or your toys.

4. Sex toys come in a mind-boggling array of types, so look for a place to buy one that either allows you to pick them up and turn them on or a website or catalog that describes them in-depth and helps you choose what's right for you. Then, be prepared to do some experimenting, giggle a little, and figure out all the different ways your toy can help you have the sex life you desire.[2]

Ellen Barnard, MSSW, is a sex educator, activist, and co-owner of A Woman's Touch Sexuality Resource Center in Madison, Wisconsin (www.awomanstouchonline.com).

I explored sex-toy stores in New York City on a recent visit. (Hey, it's a tough job, but somebody's got to do it!) I found Eve's Garden (www.evesgarden.com) discreetly situated in a midtown office building. In the lobby, there's no clue what hides behind closed doors on the twelfth floor. But a dozen flights up are shelves of vibrators, dildos, books, and novelties to decorate, stimulate, or amuse yourself. "How do people find you?" I ask the saleswoman. Women tell each other or find the store on the Internet, and some are referred by their physicians, she says.

Babeland has a store in Seattle and three more in New York. I visit the one on Mercer Street in Manhattan. The interior is bright red and yellow, playfully conveying the message that sex is fun. Toy after toy invites you to touch and turn it on. I examine vibrators in the shapes of rubber duckies, bath sponges, lipsticks, beavers, sea lions, foxes, rabbits, bears, and penises of all shapes, sizes, and colors. There are dildos built for two and a vibrator that plugs into the USB port of your computer.

A sign answers a question I've always had (but never thought to ask): "Rabbit ears? Fish tails? Funny faces? Why do some sex toys look so funny? Many of these toys were designed in Japan. For years, it was forbidden to sell vibrators for sexual purposes in Japan, so they were marketed as 'toys' and featured more whimsical designs. That's changed somewhat, but people have come to love the funny shapes and designs, and now sex-toy manufacturers from all over the world mimic these tickly designs."

See the Resources section in the Appendix for addresses and websites of all neighborhood and online sex shops mentioned in this chapter, and please send your personal favorite to joan@joanprice.com for the next edition.

CHAPTER 10

Staying Sexy without a Partner

The things that stop you having sex with age are the same as those that stop you riding a bicycle (bad health, thinking it looks silly, no bicycle). . . . The important thing is never drop sex for any long period—keep yourself going solo if you don't for the time being have a partner.

—Alex Comfort in *The Joy of Sex*[1]

Hindsight Doesn't Require Bifocals

The summer after Accident #1 (see Chapter 4, "The Bodies We Live In," to read about my two car accidents), I was thirty-four and not in a relationship. I felt greedy about grabbing some pleasure from this body that had been subjected to so much pain. I went to dances and singles' events, answered personal ads, and even propositioned casual male friends, to no avail.

I fretted that men were turned off by my limp—I used a cane, though I left it at the table when I went onto the dance floor, where I mostly jumped around on one leg.

Looking back, I'm sure (and embarrassed to admit) that the men I pursued were turned off by my intensity and desperation, not my limp. I longed for a man's touch, warmth, scent. I sought sex for much more than physical pleasure—I needed a release of pent-up anxiety and reassurance that I was still desirable. I radiated neediness.

There's nothing less sexy than desperation. It has a smell that walks in ahead of the person and signals, "Ick, run from this one!" to potential partners. I knew this—I had recognized (and run from) men who oozed desperation in the past. But I didn't know what to do about it.

So I decided I needed to work on myself, inside and out. I worked on my physical strength. I discovered that I could bicycle before I could walk, my right leg basically along for the ride while my left leg did the pedaling for both. (This worked fine as long as I didn't have to stop, because once I dismounted the only way to get back on was to find a pole or a fence to steady myself.) I also journaled and worked on my emotional resilience after this experience of powerlessness. I drew closer to friends. I bought pretty lingerie to make me feel sexy and to remind me that my skin was a world of sensation and delight, more than a bag of broken bones decorated with stitches. I liked knowing that I had a secret: lace and silk caressing my tender parts under my jeans.

And I danced with abandon, celebrating the parts of my body that worked and the adrenaline rush that kept my injuries from screaming until I stopped.

I don't know if it was the lingerie, the change in attitude, or the new enjoyment of my body as a source of pleasure rather than pain and neediness, but eventually, as I got comfortable in my body again and could focus on what I had to give rather than what I wanted to get, men stopped running away from me.

Aural Sex

Sweet Talker, sixty-five, is without a partner and celibate, but she has sex all day long—on the phone. Sweet Talker is a "phone sex goddess," as she calls herself. Here's her story:

> *I do phone sex, talk trash, and counsel men on the telephone. It works for me—and pays well, too!*
>
> *In the 1980s, I was raising my two sons solo and commuting back and forth everyday to a job I hated. I needed something that would allow me to work either closer to or from home. I came across an ad that read: "Conversationalist, Adult Talk—Work from Home!" I called. Ms. X said I had a lovely voice, and could I stop by for an interview?*
>
> *There were several desks with phones ringing, and women called "dispatchers" were answering them. Ms. X asked if I*

Sexually Seasoned Women Speak about Fulfillment without a Sexual Partner

Although I'm alone, I have a very full and exciting life. As Ellen Burstyn said, "What a lovely surprise to finally discover how unlonely being alone can be." I have met some wonderful people who have led me to adventures and opportunities to learn new things, which I might never have experienced if I had been "attached." *(Jill, 64)*

I do not have a partner or boyfriend. There are a few who would be interested in a sexual affair, but I don't want that without a long-term commitment or marriage. I don't know if I want either. I enjoy my male friends and get my hugs at the dances. I do miss the companionship, though. *(Jaime, 73)*

I am concerned about how to keep sexually fit and not lower my standards for an intimate partner. This is a dilemma—I have men friends and ex-lovers who would serve me in that way if I wanted this. But I really need to love a person's company—his in-the-moment presence—in order to want to be sexual. *(Bess, 63)*

---

had any experience, and I said, "Experience in what, talking?" We laughed, and she handed me a tape player. "Listen to this conversation between a client and the phone actress."

I listened and could feel my face getting red and hot from embarrassment. I told Ms. X the truth, that this was

I'm dating a man, but we don't have sex. I wish he would be more explicit about how he feels about me. Sometimes he gives me that look that says he'd like to gobble me up, but he doesn't express it. I wish he would. Maybe I'll bring it up myself. What we have is fine, though—it's nice to have companionship for dinner and dancing. *(Matilda, 78)*

So many women have such disappointing sex lives that they're relieved not to have a partner anymore. They don't want to get to a vulnerable, intimate place. They say, "Hypothetically, I know it would be wonderful to be in a satisfying relationship—on the other hand, I don't want to risk getting hurt again." They do a cost/benefit analysis. The benefits seem pretty remote, and the costs are really high. Sex gets tied up in a bundle with everything else. It takes a lot of work to be in a relationship. *(Nina, 67)*

Last October, when I began to think about dating again after twelve years of intentional retreat into my cave, I sent myself this email, which remains on my computer and always will: "You are loved, you are a wonderful woman, you are a sexy, smart, helpful, lovely creature, full of life in your gratitude for all you have and all of life. Life is good." *(Claire, 66)*

filth, not at all sexy to me. I said, "That's not what men want women to talk like, is it?"

She said, "Not for you, huh? Too bad. You have a very hot voice."

I asked if she would allow me to work for a week for free just to see what I could do, doing it "my way."

I went home, and my first of many calls came in. Two days later, Ms. X called to tell me I was on the payroll and to keep up the good work.

That was in 1985, and I have worked for four companies since then. I worked for one for eleven years and even had insurance and full benefits while working comfortably from my own home.

Now I am an independent "phone actress" or "phone fantasist." I talk sex to thousands upon thousands of men for money, lots of money. I have received countless gifts of lingerie, jewelry, flowers, and cold, hard cash, all from men who fall in love with my characters. I use fake names, depending on if I am the silly, young, nymphet nude dancer, Tracy, or the sophisticated sensual dominatrix, Mistress Melinda. I play many parts.

We all use models' pictures and fake names to keep our identities confidential. Many of these men want to meet me, but I say, "No, it's against the rules." After a while they move on, only to be replaced by many more. There is no shortage of men who want someone to hang on their every word and to think they are all the things they believe in their minds they are: handsome, virile, smart, sexy, and oh so desirable.

Phone sex is lies, lies, and more lies. The men lie to us, and we in turn lie right back. Do they believe us? Who knows, who cares, as long as they keep calling?

Some women begin to believe their own hype and agree to meet a man, only to be disappointed. Several girls I know actually married their callers—all but one has ended in divorce. Me, I'm still blissfully solo by choice, and still talking trash from the comfort of my own home, working whatever hours I want. I feel lucky to be able to earn a good living doing something I enjoy.

I am a single, independent lady, and a mother, a mother-in-law, and a grandmother. My kids have always known I talk to men for my job. I am not ashamed of what I do—after all, it's what I do, not who I am.

My character has never aged and remains a twenty-nine-year-old, gorgeous model. I, on the other hand, have aged gracefully and am still a beauty on the backside of sixty. The experience I have in this crazy business makes me one of the best in the world, and that's no lie. I spin slow, descriptive stories of fantasy, painting pictures in the men's minds, which they eat up, becoming extremely aroused.

In my personal life, I am celibate by choice because of HIV. Sex is dangerous and feels too risky. I don't want to die for an urge. When I was younger, even in my forties, I never thought about anything but the regular diseases, and then I didn't worry much about them. Heck, if you caught something (I never did), all you needed was a shot, but not anymore. Several of my older women friends thought because they were into menopause they didn't need to use condoms since they couldn't get pregnant. Now they are HIV positive.

I think getting horny and being able to satisfy that urge is exciting. I have heard that older women lose the desire and dry up. Not me, I still love sex, and you could call me "Juicy Lucy" wet-wise. I do what I call "tickling my fancy," sometimes with a vibrator. I don't trust most men, but I still hope one day to find the right companion for me.

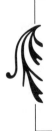

> *Forget about the mind. The clitoris is a terrible thing to waste.*
> —Lisa Kogan, writer for *O, The Oprah Magazine*

Solo Self-Pleasure:
Being Your Own Best Sex Partner

Personally, I don't like the word "masturbate." It sounds so harsh and masculine with all those hard consonants. The word has a pounding sound to it—nothing like the rhythmic tickling and rubbing that women do. I think we women need a softer, gentler word for what we do. Self-pleasure has a nice ring to it.

I read the words of the women who speak so lovingly about their own self-pleasuring, and I wish I had done that differently when I was unpartnered. I probably would have enjoyed my single years more if I had self-pleasured as a ritual rather than just getting it over with. I plugged in my vibrator for solitary sex when I needed a release of pent-up frustration so I could go about my day.

Although it was easy to give myself an orgasm that way, it was only partly satisfying. I missed the warm touch of a partner, and plastic playthings don't cuddle very well afterward. I only did it when I needed a release or worried that I'd do something stupid (like pick up the wrong man) if I didn't dull my sexual urges. I didn't build up to it, or take pleasure in it, like some of the women I interviewed. I wish now that I had. I learn so much from these women!

Touch Me, Please

The hardest part for me about being without a sex partner during my long periods of singledom was not being touched. My skin and my mind hungered for it. Fortunately, I had friends who liked to hug, and I burrowed into their arms at every opportunity.

I also found social dancing to be a wonderful source of respectful, nonsexual touching that went a long way toward filling that need. I went to dances at least twice a week and freely asked men to dance rather than waiting for them to ask me. I discovered which partners were good dancers and good leaders, which ones flirted appealingly, and which ones felt and smelled nice. If someone turned out to be a bad choice—showed off rather than danced *with* me, reeked of alcohol or old sweat, or looked over my head for younger, prettier women—well, it was just two minutes of my life. Most of the time, though, dancing gave me the immense pleasure of being in men's arms—and I became a pretty good dancer!

I sometimes got therapeutic massages during my sexless times. I recommend massage, though I don't recommend what I did: I was so stifled with unexpressed desire, so hungry for touch on the parts of my body that were skipped during a professional massage, that I seduced two of my massage practitioners.

In both cases, I was the one to communicate wordlessly that I was open (so to speak) to the massage going further. Both were kind and gentle men who loved giving pleasure with their hands. Both were surprised that they let themselves respond to the sexual feelings in the air (they both said they had never let that happen before), and at first they felt guilty that our affairs had begun on the massage table. One affair lasted for several months, and the other, casually, for several years.

Sexually Seasoned Women Speak about Solo Sex

Here's how I masturbate. It's a real performance-art kind of thing. I put on some music, like Chet Baker's good, slinky jazz. I dress myself carefully in a black lace teddy. I arrange two or three mirrors. I get out some coconut oil. I pretend I am someone else enjoying watching the person I see in the mirrors. I speak to her. I tell her how good she looks and appreciate her beauty and willingness to do what I say. There's also an element of control and domination. I tell her what to do, and then praise her for it. I touch my breasts, especially the nipples. I get very close to the mirror with my pussy and praise its beauty. I try to prolong it, but usually I come very quickly. *(Rachel, 62)*

When I was single and my grown son was out of the house, I discovered sex with myself in a wonderful way. I had a mad, passionate, love affair with myself. I got fabulous lingerie and bought myself champagne. It was just me and a vibrator. Some days, nobody else can do it like you. *(Monica, 60)*

I used to masturbate until I was almost raw, getting almost mad at myself because I couldn't make myself come. That was when I was in my thirties and forties. Now it's a snap. I know that I need a lot of lubrication and make sure my bottle is handy. *(Aurora, 60)*

I left my last relationship about twelve years ago and wanted to be a hermit. I continued to be sexual with myself and got pretty wonderful results with that method. When I felt sexual, I made love to myself, just like I comforted myself as a kid. Now I'm turned on all the time. *(Claire, 66)*

I should masturbate, but I find it creates more loneliness. I'd rather not think about it. When I do, I use videos. Masturbating is physically satisfying, but emotionally it brings up feelings I don't want. I have the ability to just deaden my sex drive until something *(or someone)* sparks it. *(Erica, 62)*

I was maybe sixty-five before I ever did it. I was talking with a girlfriend who was between relationships, and she said she masturbated. I never even thought of such a thing. My first time, I knew just where to go. I tried it with the jets in the hot tub, and I found the right spot. It was the best sex I ever had! I was never one to have a climax easily with men. By the time I got close, they were already done. I get more climaxes this way than I ever did with a man. *(Jaime, 73)*

I enjoy solo sex, especially when I'm alone for extended periods of time. Listening to soothing music, thinking about it ahead of time, wearing tight-fitting clothes, and moving around to the music in them in front of a mirror is quite stimulating to me. *(Ulla, 61)*

Sometimes I masturbate—what else can you do? It's better than going out and picking up people. My drive is still strong. *(Matilda, 78)*

Vaginal Rejuvenation & Health

If time is passing between periods of intimacy and penetrative sex, you should keep your vagina tuned up and healthy. Myrtle Wilhite, MD, MS, and co-owner of A Woman's Touch Sexuality Resource Center in Madison, Wisconsin, offers the following tips for genital health:

External Moisturizing and Massage: Increase the suppleness and blood circulation of the skin of your vulva and vagina with a five- to ten-minute massage with a moisturizing sexual lubricant like Liquid Silk, a water-based lotion that will soak in and moisturize your skin, won't get sticky, and will help you massage with very little friction.

Push into the skin with circular strokes, and massage what's underneath the skin rather than brushing across the skin. Include the inner lips, the hood of the clitoris, the head of the clitoris, and the perineum.

To complete your external massage, massage into the opening of the vaginal canal, using the same circular strokes. The massage itself does not need to be self-sexual in any way, but if that is comfortable for you, by all means explore these sensations.

Internal Vaginal Massage: To massage inside your vaginal canal, we suggest using a Lucite dildo, which is very smooth and will not cause friction or tearing. Choose your size based upon how many fingers you can comfortably insert into the opening of your vagina.

After a session of external vulva massage, apply the same massage to the inner surfaces of your vagina with your dildo, with lubricant applied on both skin and dildo. Rather than pushing the dildo in and out, use a circular massage movement. You are increasing skin flexibility so that your body can adjust to comfortable sexual penetration if you choose it.

You might also choose to use a slim vibrator for massaging the vaginal walls. Coat it in Liquid Silk, and then insert it gently. Turn it on, and let it run for about five minutes. You don't need to move it around, just lie there and let it do its work.

Orgasm: For women who stop having orgasms, the blood vessels literally can get out of shape, preventing future orgasms. If you are able to bring yourself to orgasm, do so at least once a week for the rest of your life. (Seriously.) This is preventive maintenance of your body.

Kegel Relaxation: Kegels increase both the strength and flexibility of your pelvic-floor muscles. Pay attention to the relaxation and deep-breath part of the exercise. Learning to relax your pelvic floor will help you to avoid tensing up before penetration. (See Chapter 6, "Fitness and Exercise: Our Bodies, Ourselves, Our Sex Lives," for Dr. Wilhite's tips for perfect Kegels.)[2]

Doctor's Orders

"Genital atrophy" is a scary phrase. It's common in postmeno-pausal women after discontinuing HRT, according to a 2005 observational study.[3] Murray Freedman, MD, a clinical professor of OBGYN at the Medical College of Georgia, Augusta, and an expert in genital atrophy in postmenopausal women, addressed a medical conference to suggest that doctors recommend inter-course at least once a week to their postmenopausal patients to help maintain tissue integrity by dilation and increased genital blood flow. "It's a use-it-or-lose-it phenomenon," he explained.

Dr. Freedman suggested that women without a male part-ner be counseled to use topical estrogen and a vibrator and to have periodic orgasms. "This will maintain a normal, healthy vagina," he said.

"At what age would you like your genitalia to begin shrink-ing?" he challenged male physicians who never bring up the sub-ject of sexuality with their postmenopausal patients.

Juicy Is an Attitude

Haven't you noticed that when you're getting plenty of sex, peo-ple are attracted to you as if you were oozing irresistible come-hithers, while when you're desperate for sex or a relationship, you might as well be wearing a sign that says, "I have a stinky, fatal disease—stay far away"?

Being sexually juicy doesn't depend on the flow of our vaginal secretions or the presence of a partner in our life but on physical and emotional well-being, mental attitude, and love of sensuality.

We can feel and look sexy and attractive, whether we're in a relationship or not. Looking good has nothing to do with whether our thighs are tight or dimply, our breasts perky or floppy, our face unlined or road-mapped. Any partner who would judge us this way would be much too superficial for a relationship at this stage of our lives, anyway. Sexiness is how we feel about ourselves and how we present ourselves to the world, with or without a partner.

We are lively and sexy when we live our lives fully, doing the activities that keep us energetic, creative, and happy whether we're accompanied by a lover or not. The more we strut our beautiful stuff with confidence, the more others are attracted to us.

CHAPTER 11

Hunting Ground: In the Dating Game Again (or Still)

Cold Flashes

After menopause, I experienced dry spells socially as well as internally. There was a long, dark period that lasted years, when I didn't know if I'd ever attract men again. When I was younger, I'd smile and make eye contact with a man, and a few minutes or hours of conversation later, we'd make a date. If I wanted to go to bed with someone, I could almost always count on him being willing.

But as I got into my late forties and fifties, paddling my way into the dating scene after a breakup of a long-term relationship, I discovered that my social world had dried up—along with my ability to attract men who attracted me. I would smile at a man who looked appealing or interesting, and he would look right past me. I was invisible.

Sometimes I would succeed in engaging a man in conversation, but his eyes would roam the room, as if looking for better luck. Sure enough, a young woman whose firm skin and open-to-there clothing screamed "Young and hot!" would appear, and he'd be off.

I understood it: I even wrote a feature article for *Men's Fitness* magazine explaining lust and how men, especially young men, are hardwired to spread their seed and propagate (despite carrying condoms), so they are attracted to women who advertise their fertility. And we all know about the middle-aged man's crisis, when a younger woman is a neon sign blinking, "I'm with Mr. Virile-and-Successful here."

So, where does that leave us? Many best-selling books, films, and TV shows have examined our predicament, but usually with either ridicule or loathing. We seldom find examples of the zesty, sexy, middle- and older-aged women that we know ourselves to be!

Love Dances In

When I was trying so hard to meet men, my friends would tell me, "Why are you line dancing? You won't meet men line

Sexually Seasoned Women Speak about the Challenges of Finding a Partner

Sex after sixty would be great if I could find the right man. Sex before sixty was great, so I'm sure it would be even better now because I feel more secure. I have met and dated a number of men since my divorce fifteen years ago. At first, I "needed" to have a male in my life. I joined a bowling team and a singles group, took dance classes, golf lessons, auto-repair classes, and wine-tasting classes, and joined hiking groups. But the single men I met wanted a mother, nurse, housekeeper, or cook—or all of these! I'm done with all that. I want a fun-loving, active, and fit man who is ready to explore travel opportunities with me, such as archaeological digs, volunteer environmental work trips, and backpacking. I want someone who will travel off the beaten track with me. *(Jill, 64)*

Lesbians are famous for meeting, falling in love, crawling in bed, moving in, and moving out! *(Claire, 66)*

Looking for love as an older woman can be deflating to the ego. The men tend to flock to the younger women, and one has to have a strong stomach to stay with it. More than once, I drove home from a dance crying because the men my age were interested in women ten or more years younger. I don't cry on the way home anymore, but it took quite a while to develop friends and men who I know like to dance with me. *(Melanie, 64)*

It's harder to find a great relationship when you're older. Here I am—I look younger than I am, I've been involved in many interesting things, and I'm outgoing, funny, and bright. And I can't get nothing! *(Nina, 67)*

I got divorced from my third husband at sixty-one and haven't dated since except to go to bingo, line dancing, bowling, a writers group and the community pool. I haven't actively looked for love. My challenge is that I am sixty-five but look closer to forty-something. Younger men hit on me and are shocked when I prove my age to them. They say I'm too pretty, I don't have enough wrinkles, and I'm too active to be that old. I never want to be any man's old lady, so the younger ones don't work for my taste. The older men are usually not much fun—they don't have enough energy and are boring. I'm still looking! *(Catherine, 65)*

I'm sixty-two and could use a lift in a lot of places, but I'm still cute and charming. If you're single, having sex after sixty is easy. Finding a relationship is not. I was a big Internet dater. Initially, it was great. I met a lot of men, had sex with a lot of men, and had a mad, passionate affair with one. Then it got really old. I'd go out on dates, and they'd be duds. If I were a man, I'd have lots of opportunities. I know a sixty-two-year-old guy who put up a profile and was inundated with responses—mostly from terrific women. He's now dating (and having sex with) a few of them and is bemoaning the fact that he just can't say no. What a problem! I'm attracting the bottom-feeders myself. *(Erica, 62)*

continued on the next page

continued from page 161

I can tell you that my youthful, brash "come-on" techniques no longer feel right. I dread the thought of rejection, which I used to take in stride—some you win, some you lose. I don't want to be seen as a "dirty old woman," so I don't come on to guys in any serious way. I just flirt, which comes naturally to me. *(Rachel, 62)*

I look at some of the women my age, and they don't push themselves. I see women at dances sitting there, with a man sitting two seats away, and they don't ask him to dance. I do. I wouldn't do that when I was younger, but I do now. I'm much more outgoing than when I was younger. I get a lot of responses I never got before and more people asking me out. A lot of women think, This is it, and they don't even want to try. *(Matilda, 78)*

I am too proud to risk the rejection. Plus, I'm a Goddess worshipper, and I tell Her, "If you want me to have a man, you put him in my pathway. I'm not going out trolling." I just go along through the world being an attractive and sexy human being not on the make. *(Rachel, 62)*

dancing." After years of teaching early-morning aerobics classes, I was now teaching evening line-dance classes, and I loved it. But gosh, men were in short supply there. Maybe I should take an auto-mechanics class. *Not!*

The day that Robert walked into my line-dance class, my hormones thought they were twenty years old again. His smile, fit body, and grace of movement caught my eye immediately.

Then, when he started to dance, his years of tap, modern dance, and ballet training were revealed in every movement, and I was lost at sea. His nimble feet, muscled thighs, and sensually mobile hips commanded my attention. I wanted to touch the inviting curl of chest hair that peeked through the open top buttons of his shirt. I met his dazzling blue eyes and pretended to breathe. For the rest of the evening, I kept losing my place in the dance I was teaching because I couldn't take my eyes off him.

Robert kept coming to class and danced into my heart. I tried to engage him in conversation after class occasionally, and he responded almost warily, answering me but not giving me any signals that my attentions were welcomed or reciprocated. I wondered, *Is he gay? Attached? Or simply not interested in me?*

I started inviting him for walks after class, which he accepted. We talked, but never very personally. I told him about the Internet health book I was writing, and he told me about his art and the English gardens of his travels. There was no touching, no eyes locking, no double entendres, no intimate details revealed.

We choreographed a line dance together, which felt extraordinarily intimate to me. We were using our bodies to communicate and showing each other movements, which was very sexy. But the harder I tried to push to the next stage, the faster he retreated.

We laugh now about how long it took before he returned my interest—nine months! Finally, I sent him a daring email:

> *Let me tell you something I haven't shared verbally, though you probably sense it from the unspoken signals. I am deliciously attracted to you. That doesn't mean we have to act on it, though if you kissed me, I'd kiss you back.*

Sometimes when I watch you dance, I wonder what it would be like to hold you—without footwork.

I have no idea if the attraction is mutual—and if it isn't, it won't affect our growing friendship in any way. (But it would be nice if you'd tell me bluntly how you're reacting to this news, now that I've spilled this to you!)

Do I say more, or delete what I said? Do I reassure you that you don't have to feel the same way? You can say, "That's flattering, but no, it's not a direction I want to go," and I won't bring it up again, nor will it affect my enjoyment of you. The one thing that would make me feel bad is if you wanted to back off and stop dancing with me!

How much power that "Send" button has now!

Robert responded that he was attracted to me, too, and he admired my courage in writing to him—but he didn't feel the need to rush things.

Rush things? Nine months?

"I wanted to get to know you first," he said later. And I—whose motto used to be "The only problem with instant gratification is that it takes too long!"—waited for him to be ready.

Well, I sort of waited. Two weeks later, we took a walk after class, and I propositioned him.

He turned me down.

"I don't get involved in sex casually," he told me. He wanted a spiritual connection first. He had been celibate for four years, which he said was not a problem for him. His words and looks were kind, and I did not feel rejected. This was a man worth waiting for.

I was surprised by an email from Robert later that night. He had changed his mind:

If your interest is in having a sexual relationship, I would be open to discussing this further. It wouldn't take a whole lot of discussion. It could be fun. But you must keep in mind that I am sometimes a young person in an old body and sometimes an old person in an old body. In any case, I see you as being understanding of whatever dimensions of body and/or spirit you may want to explore with me. It's been a while for the body parts. It may be about time.

We made a date to take a walk after the next dance class and discuss what to do next. We strolled under the full moon, not touching, and then stopped at a park bench. There we shared our first kiss. And our second. Third. Twentieth. We necked and petted like teenagers, the silver moonlight spotlighting our excitement. Then we made a plan to spend the following Saturday at his house and explore the next dimension of our relationship.

We didn't know that we would fall in love. But we did. That was four years ago as I write this, and we've been a committed couple ever since. In November 2004, we became engaged. Robert is the man I've been seeking my whole life and finally met at age fifty-seven. It is my great privilege to love him.

Joanna, Sixty-one, Tells of Meeting Her Husband Online

After eight years in a relationship that was going nowhere, but which I continued because of the regular sex, I dumped my boyfriend and started looking on the Internet. I was in my late fifties. I joined twelve online services. I was surprised by how many men out there were interested in me, and also by how many high-quality men there were. Altogether, I got to know about six nice guys through online dating.

One of the online services I joined let me post my profile for free, but a membership fee was required in order to read any received messages. I waited until I had notice that I'd received a letter from "Pete." I looked up his profile and was blown away. This handsome professor seemed to be everything I had dreamed of: intellectual, funny, and an academic. I paid $60 to join the service and dropped Pete a line. He phoned right away. In our conversation, we discovered that we had an amazing number of things in common. He told me that he had to go out of the country for two weeks but would get back to me as soon as he returned.

The next day, I received another letter from a member who had posted no profile. In my experience with the dating services, I had learned to avoid the no-profile guys, but I decided to read his letter anyway.

The letter was just wonderful! It came from a retired businessman who was now a small-business entrepreneur. His letter bubbled with personality. It felt as if it had come from an old friend. And, more amazing, he also lived in my hometown. He phoned me, and we talked for two hours, until my portable phone ran out of batteries. We arranged to meet for brunch the next morning.

As I started toward the restaurant where we were to meet, I thought to myself, "My whole life is about to *change." I walked in, and Gordon was sitting in the corner, reading the paper. I knew him immediately.*

We had a wonderful brunch, and I invited him to come home with me to watch a baseball game. Then I invited him to stay for the evening—and the night.

The next day, I closed my account with all the dating services and emailed Pete that I had found someone else. Two weeks later, Gordon and I decided to get married. The wedding was seven months to the day from when we met. We've been married for two years.

Claire's Story: Finding True Love Online

I started online dating five months ago. The first week or two, I had so many women contacting me that I had to make a flow chart—who should I write back to? It made me feel I was still a sexual person.

The woman I'm in love with now was the only one who mentioned sex in her profile, as I did. She said, "Must have a healthy libido." I said, "Must enjoy sexual pleasure." I realized I can ask for what I want from another woman. I can say that if you're not interested in being sexual, I'm not interested in going any further. Life is getting short here, and I've got to go for it. A lot of younger lesbians wrote, "I'm interested in a mature older woman." I wrote back, "So am I. Good luck to you."

I fell in love with K before we saw each other physically. So when we did see each other, we had all the other questions pretty much answered and spent a weekend making

Sexually Seasoned Women Speak about Fertile Hunting Grounds

I've used every method and resource: singles ads locally and also in French singles papers when I was living in France, singles groups and activities like Sierra Singles, vacations at Club Med, giving interesting parties and holding "salons" at my home and asking people to bring available single men, and traveling all over the world on my own and being open to meeting men and having love affairs. *(Phoebe, 64)*

There are younger lesbians who are attracted to me at sixty-six, with my share of wrinkles. It wouldn't matter because my personality is more important to them. There are others who want someone who looks good on their arm. I feared that when I went online with my picture. But that's not what I found. There are so many older women looking for each other with their hearts more than their eyes. *(Claire, 66)*

blissful love, reading poems to each other, and dancing to Etta James's "At Last."

We have been making love online ever since. She will be here soon for a week. I bet this will be the most interesting little mobile home in this senior mobile-home park. Great energy will be radiating out into the world.

I have decided to relocate to be with my love. It's been interesting to tell people and watch them freak out. "So soon? Don't you think you should wait a year?"

I met my companion of fifteen years at a senior dance when I was sixty-two. I had a date with somebody else. When I danced with him, the electricity was there. That started it. I had not had an orgasm with anybody for a long time, and with him, I did. It wasn't anything he did; it was the electricity between us. *(Matilda, 78)*

I took up activities that I enjoyed: environmental clubs, hiking and biking groups, and singles groups at churches. I joined some dance clubs and began going to the dances. I enrolled in an expensive dating club, and that was totally a waste of money. One could read biographical information and see a picture and a video. I only had one response to my picks, and it was from a man eight years younger. We had a five-month relationship—we had great sex, but he was an alcoholic. I finally decided it wasn't worth it. *(Melanie, 64)*

Love finds me. I don't do the singles scene, and I don't do the Internet. I just live my life, and they find me. I meet lots of men who like me. I discriminate on the criteria of passion and fun. *(Bess, 63)*

My response is, "Hey, wake up, she's sixty-one, I'm sixty-six. What the hell do we want to wait for—to get older?"

Looking for Love in All the Right Places

As a younger woman, I frequented singles activity groups and discussions, placed and answered personal ads, attended singles parties and dances, danced in bars (nursing one mineral water all evening), and went on plenty of blind dates. I was rewarded with lots of dates and both short-term and long-term relationships,

Around the Block: Erotic Adventures of Single Sexually Seasoned Women

I met this Israeli guy through the Internet. He was extremely good looking. We had a first date in Manhattan, and we made out madly in Riverside Park. Then I invited him to visit me. Turns out he was into rough sex. He literally ripped off my clothes, and we had sex instantly. I really enjoyed it, having such a great-looking guy desire me passionately. But once was enough. After that, I didn't like being mauled. I told him it wasn't what I was into, and he went away. *(Erica, 62)*

Recently, while camping on the Libyan desert during Ramadan, our security guard, an attractive man around thirty years old, fell deeply in lust for me. The night Ramadan ended, he came to my tent, and we masturbated each other to orgasm. *(Phoebe, 64)*

At age sixty, I had a neighbor in his seventies who was a sex fiend. I went with him for about two years. He wanted sex all the time, even though he had to take shots to get an erection. When he wasn't here, he would call me for phone sex. But he only wanted to satisfy himself—he didn't care about my satisfaction. When I was at his house, he would make sure I didn't leave anything behind, even a hairpin. After a while, I got smart. He was seeing other women. Then I found out he was getting married, and then he died. *(Matilda, 78)*

I had an affair when I turned sixty. I went to a conference for lesbians. I was on a panel. When I stepped down from the podium, a videographer came up and asked if she could do a private interview. Our eyes met—we both went crazy. We began a six-month affair. She was very sexual, and she had a bag of sex toys she brought when she came to visit. But she turned out to be too controlling in sex. I didn't like it—I prefer a gentler approach to having my body touched. If you grew up with humiliation and violence, you don't need to play games to find out what it feels like. *(Claire, 66)*

When my libido resurfaced after menopause, I signed up with a swingers website. Saying that you are a swinger rather than that you are looking for sex seems to get a more considerate type of male. I met two men who were really great—one was fifty and the other twenty-five. I arranged to meet both of them at a local saloon. The bartender knew what I was doing. She almost drooled over the younger guy. His handle was "handsomeandhorny," and he was both. *(Kaycee, 66)*

A Male's Perspective on Internet Dating

Ralph, seventy, is a single man seeking a meaningful relationship. He shares his male perspective on older singles looking for love through online dating:

There are good women and good men on the Internet. You write emails back and forth and develop confidence. Then you go for coffee. When I go for coffee with a lady, I interview her, and I'm sure she does this, too. It's fine for either of us to say, "We're not a match." There's no sense wasting our time. If the coffee date is good, we go for a movie, and I try to expand the relationship.

If she has a good heart and we talk easily, things flow. I think, Oh, man, I could easily spend hours talking with this lady. If she has wrinkles or she's heavy but she has a good heart, I think there's something to work on. I've been susceptible to beautiful women, but I hate myself when that happens.

I'm a touchy guy. I like a woman who doesn't mind physical contact, like hugging and touching me on the arm when she says hello. Some women won't put out their hands, even for a handshake. We men are the ones doing the reaching out and taking the risk of rejection. I might touch her elbow to see if that's acceptable.

She has to have a nice personality, and we have to have chemistry. If that's not there, forget it. I'm seventy, and I don't have too many more years to find the right woman. It's the same for older women.

casual and serious. At the time, I felt I was putting a lot of energy into meeting men and kissing too many frogs. In retrospect, I had it easy: I was a young, outgoing, attractive woman.

As a woman over fifty, I found the whole dating scene much more frustrating. Again, I placed and answered personal ads, and this time, I also used online ads. I had lots of first dates this way, but I found that although the flurry of emails or phone calls had been promising, once I met the person, the chemistry just wasn't there. I know that physical attraction can develop over time if the mind and heart connections are there—this has happened to me in the past—but these men made my expectations drop into my sneakers when I saw them. No way, sorry.

I decided it would be more fruitful to go to events where men with my interests were likely to go, and where I could see if the chemistry had a fighting chance before pursuing anything.

I mainly went to dances, choosing alcohol-free venues (I had no interest in meeting men who liked to meet women in bars or who needed to fortify themselves with alcohol in order to dance). Dancing was—and is—a great love of mine, and since it was important to me that my partner be a dancer, this was the most logical path.

Some women join outdoor activities groups, and others get involved in political or community action organizations, join discussion groups, or volunteer for good causes. I think the best way to meet the partner who will suit you is to do what you love to do and go places and participate in activities where your potential partner would be if his or her interests matched yours.

Be Careful, Please

This happened in my twenties in New York City, but it could happen at any age and in any city.

I accepted a date with a man I had met on a commuter train. We took the same train each day and often talked. Ronald was attractive, intelligent, and well dressed. I'm not saying that "well dressed" was one of my hot buttons, just that it spelled "safe" to me. When he proposed that we go out to dinner and a Broadway play, I accepted eagerly. My job teaching in an alternative high school didn't permit me such extravagance on my own, plus he seemed like a fellow I'd like to know better. My live-in boyfriend had unexpectedly left me, and while the relationship was still in limbo, I wanted to explore what else was out there.

I offer all these details to explain—not excuse—why I was so stupid.

We went to a lovely, expensive restaurant and to a popular play. Ronald accompanied me back to my apartment to "make sure I got home safely." Once inside, he refused to leave. "I spent good money on you," he said. "You owe me."

He grabbed me and slid his hands over my body. I cried, "No!" and pulled away. He strengthened his grip. He pushed me down on the couch and pinned me with his arms and legs, angry with my resistance.

My little dog, a toy fox terrier, started barking wildly. "I'll kill that mutt!" Ronald yelled, but fortunately the dog distracted him enough that I managed to get out from under him and escape. I grabbed the dog and ran into the hall, where I shouted for help. Luckily, a neighbor—a hefty man in his twenties—ran to me and protected me while ordering Ronald to leave.

Stupidly, I blamed myself and never reported Ronald to the police. Although I know this is a common reaction, I feel guilty now about leaving him free to pull this same dangerous game on the next woman. This never occurred to me at the time—I was just grateful to have escaped. From then on, I took a different commuter train and paid my own way on dates.

I learned from this to have first dates in public, inexpensive places—coffee dates or walks in a park—and not to invite men into my home until I felt comfortable with them.

Note to Readers: Try This

I run into one of my interviewees at a conference. "Still single," she tells me.

"Just wait until this book comes out," I tell her. "Then carry it around to your trolling places, and tell each man you meet, 'I'm in this book. I won't tell you which person I am, but I'm *very* interesting!'"

CHAPTER 12

Done It All— Ready to Nest

A girl can wait for the right man to come along, but, in the meantime, that doesn't mean she can't have a wonderful time with all the wrong ones.

—Cher

I was a sexual explorer in my twenties—not sure what uncharted territory I would discover, open to adventure, glorying in my newfound sexuality. At the same time, my goals were traditional:

I wanted to fall in love with the perfect man who would wrap up love, great sex, romance, intimacy, excitement, intellectual stimulation, and sensitivity all in one package. Then my wanderlust would end, I thought.

I was right—but it took me until age fifty-seven to meet him, with many wonderful men (and some not so wonderful) along the way. I had several long-term relationships, one growth-giving marriage to a wonderful man who remains my dear friend, and lots of flings.

Heating Up: Sex, Love, and Marriage

I discovered fantastic sex when I lived in Italy for three years after college, but the out-of-bed relationships didn't match the quality of the under-the-covers experience.

• Paolo, my first Italian lover, was a sensual, pleasure-giving sex partner who helped teach me to speak Italian and then didn't care about hearing my thoughts once I was able to express them.

• Marcello, my two-year lover—with whom I fantasized about staying in Florence forever—read Italian poetry to me and made love to me as if I were the most desirable woman in the world but never introduced me to his mother (with whom he still lived, as Italian men did until they married). And, I learned later, he cheated on me repeatedly, even in my own bed.

• Giuliano, my rebound lover, was a superb sex partner and a lot of fun as a companion, but he borrowed money from me and never repaid me.

I returned from Italy disillusioned but ready to reinvent my life. I had been in a country that had barely changed in pace and culture since the Renaissance, and I returned to the America of

1968—what a shock! But I adjusted quickly. I packed up my elegant wool suits in favor of jeans with embroidered patches and a macrame belt.

I fell in love with Arnie, a bearded alternative-school teacher with a warm smile and heart, songs spilling from his lips and guitar, and a fierce need to help right the wrongs of the world. At our first meeting, we talked all night and declared ourselves in love. Within weeks, we were living together, and a year and a half later, we married.

About halfway through our four-and-a-half-year marriage, Arnie and I started talking about "opening" our relationship to admit other lovers. It was the early seventies, and all around us were couples who seemed to be doing just fine having sex with their friends—singles with marrieds, marrieds with other marrieds, singles with each other's significant others. The Youngbloods's hit song "Get Together" resounded as our generation's anthem:

C'mon people now,
Smile on your brother
Ev'rybody get together
Try and love one another right now

I was attracted to another teacher at the high school where I taught. Arnie and I resolutely supported each other's autonomy and growth and felt our bond was strong enough to accept my having a sexual relationship with another person. In fact, it was. I became giddy with sexual excitement and felt "primed" when I went from an after-school tryst with my new lover to the arms of my husband. It was the best of all worlds. Arnie experimented also, sometimes staying overnight with a regular lover, sometimes frolicking with someone new. Our marriage felt alive and exciting.

It surprises me now that we did so well exploring this brave new world, but we were strong communicators, and it worked. These outside relationships added sparks to our own sexual interaction, and after they played themselves out (which they did), we were left as strongly united as before.

Until Kyle.

I fell madly in love with Kyle, despite many reasons I shouldn't have, among them that I let my marriage shatter. I left Arnie to live with Kyle. Four years later, Kyle fell in love with another woman and left me to live with her. My just desserts.

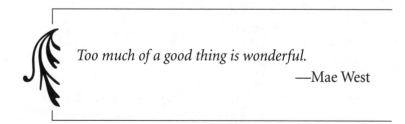

Too much of a good thing is wonderful.
—Mae West

Firing on All Cylinders: The Emancipated Woman

I went wild, enjoying multiple relationships—sometimes serially, sometimes simultaneously—from my mid-thirties to my early forties. I felt juicy and ripe, both physically and emotionally. I placed and answered personal ads, joined singles groups, and went out dancing. I lived in my own Age of Aquarius, reveling in the heady excitement of each new man. How would his

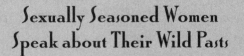

Sexually Seasoned Women
Speak about Their Wild Pasts

Of course, casual sex was much more likely to happen in my twenties. Not only was the body ready, but it was that precious window of historical time: birth control was cheap and readily available, and herpes had not reared its ugly head—not to mention there was no fear of HIV or AIDS. *(Rachel, 62)*

I was really experimental. Sandstone, multiple partners, swinging, polyamory—I tried all of it. At the same time, I was on a spiritual exploration—a student, a hippie, and a budding psychotherapist. I don't think I missed out on any opportunity. It was also a time pre-HIV, and STDs weren't too big a problem. Now, I know I was lucky to have come out of all that unscathed, but I did, and it was all a great experience. *(Tina, 61)*

I led a high-spirited sex life during my thirties. Once, I was at a party, and I realized that I had been to bed with three of the men in the room. It sent a shiver of excitement through me that I knew these men so intimately, and there they were, talking to each other casually. Another time, my roommate told me that a man had called, left his first name, and requested that I call back about the plans for our upcoming date. I had upcoming dates with two men of that same first name, and I didn't know whom to call back! More than once I had a date with one man in the afternoon and another in the evening—I felt so full of sexual energy! *(Diana, 62)*

In my twenties, I was quite wild, a hippie girl. I married twice—at ages eighteen and twenty-five—and divorced at thirty. In the first marriage, there were many lovers. We were so young, and it was the sixties, a time of free love. We thought we could just sleep with anybody. But the men were mostly just getting off on being able to sleep with the "good girls." It was degrading in many ways. I felt used. In my thirties, I pulled back from sex. Then I began to experiment with younger men who were raised in a society where women were accepted as equals. *(Monica, 60)*

I could probably write a book about my sexual escapades. I was a very busy, active lady. At age twenty-three, I started an affair with a married man twenty years older. He was cute, funny, and a fantastic dresser. I usually wouldn't have dated a married man with three children, but, you see, I knew his wife, and she was a tramp—she would go into a parked van with several men at once. Plus, she chased the guy I was dating. So I figured maybe her husband had the right to and the need for my attention. Our affair was hot and heavy and lasted for ten years. He set me up in an apartment, with no strings attached. Even after I married my second husband, I still continued the affair. *(Catherine, 65)*

continued on next page

Better Than I Ever Expected

continued from page 181

As a younger woman, I wanted sex more often—and I often masturbated a few times a day. I would have sex with inappropriate partners just to have sex. I had very few long-term relationships, and very few sexually satisfying ones. Then AIDS came along, and I had to be more careful, and I couldn't find anyone I cared about enough to get to know. *(Joanna, 61)*

Because I was told that I couldn't have sex with women, my desire became like a wild horse they tried to corral. I was in the Navy—oh, my goodness, what you have to do to find a place to be sexual with another woman when you're in the Navy. They kick you out in a hot second if you are caught. I did it under beds, in closets, in the shower, in the bushes in back of the barracks, and in the middle of the night surrounded by eighty other women sleeping— I learned to be very quiet. I would spend my whole life owning my right to be a sexual person with the women I chose. *(Claire, 66)*

After my divorce, I was a bit wild. The Catholic training had finally worn off, and I was ready for action. I had dropped out of college when I got pregnant, but then I returned after my second child was born. I divorced soon after. I had an affair with my college professor. Wearing only a raincoat, I picked him up from a night class. I had a threesome once: two women and one man. It was interesting but not something I wanted to repeat. *(Susie, 60)*

I had a very promiscuous youth and slept with hundreds of men. My life was just like the TV show *Sex and the City* except for the shoes: a single girl in New York, having a ball. I had the same girlfriends. We did the same things—we'd screw around and dish about men, being witty and clever. *(Erica, 62)*

When I was married in my twenties, my now ex-husband was very cold and naive about sex. Only after my divorce at thirty-one, at the height of the women's movement, did I learn what good sex was. From the seventies through the nineties, I was totally open to everything and had terrific lovers and sex all over the world. I had about twenty-five years of single freedom with many, many different lovers. *(Phoebe, 64)*

When I was in my thirties, I had an affair during my first marriage and experimented with some things like spanking, new variations of oral sex, and anal sex. The thrill of a secret affair seemed to add to the excitement. Using mirrors, masturbating for him, and using vibrators on each other really aroused me. Just making love in so many creative ways with a stranger was amazingly exciting. I've never enjoyed anal sex since with anyone, but this partner was so gentle and did so many other things simultaneously—he massaged my buttocks, breasts, and vagina, and used his mouth and fingers all over my body. The marriage was not good anyway, and after this affair, it crumbled completely. *(Ulla, 61)*

kisses feel? How would he look naked? How would he touch me? What noises would he make?

I never considered myself promiscuous—my definition of promiscuous: someone who has sex with many more people than I do!—I was just lucky enough to meet a batch of sexy, energetic, and attractive men who were also interested in me. So I dated around and went to bed with willing partners who shared a mutual attraction.

Most of these relationships either started as or resulted in friendship. I was not going for notches on my belt; I just enjoyed sexual variety. I was honest with my partners, and they (as far as I knew) were honest with me. I got away lucky with no STDs and just a mild case of lip herpes that surfaces once a year or so.

I entered into sexual relationships with three of the men I met in one singles discussion group—and the facilitator. Two other lovers of that era were cousins who lived together. (Once they met in my parking lot, one leaving and one arriving, and shook hands as they passed.) I preferred younger men at the time—I liked their energy, their open-mindedness, and their absence of stereotypes about women. I found older men stodgy and closed-minded. (How wrong I was, I was still to discover!)

Once, a bunch of women friends and I placed a personal ad that started, "Twelve lively women wonder if the men we are seeking exist. . . ." We got more than a hundred responses and exchanged grocery bags filled with their letters in order to read them all. We made a chart so we could decide who would answer which letters. I met two lovers that way.

Many of these relationships went on for months, and some developed into affectionate friendships that lasted long after the sex stopped. I met my lifelong best male friend during that time.

Intellectually, I would have liked to have been an equal-opportunity adventurer and experimented with women, too—but biologically, my hardwiring just didn't entice me to go there. I loved women as friends, but my sex drive catapulted me to men exclusively. I just wasn't turned on sexually by female bodies. I think we're each somewhere on a biologically determined continuum between exclusively heterosexual and exclusively homosexual, and that placement determines whether we're turned on by the opposite gender, our own gender, or some proportion of both.

Two Plus One Equals Three

I tried threesomes three different times. In each case, I was already enjoying sex with both men independently and thought it would be thrilling to experience them together. They knew and liked each other (though had not sexually experimented with each other) and were willing, mainly to please me.

As much as sex with two men had been a constant fantasy of mine, the reality was disappointing. The visual experience was great, but in each case, I either didn't orgasm or had a really hard time getting there because there was too much going on. I couldn't focus enough to come. Even navigating was challenging: there were all these elbows and knees everywhere. It was more weird than exciting. But I have no regrets—I wanted to experience this, and I did.

As embarrassing as some of these admissions are, I'm not at all sorry that I had any of these experiences. Having multiple relationships was exhilarating. They helped me figure out just what I did and didn't want from a relationship.

Sexually Seasoned Women Reminisce about Special Past Lovers

She was a very imaginative woman in bed and out. She had an upstairs apartment, and she attached a rack of those bells that you would find on an ice cream cart to a string outside her apartment, which hung down to a secret spot that only I knew about. When I came to see her, I would "ring her bells," as she put it. She was an amazingly comfortable and enjoyable person to have fun with. We made love in haylofts we found along country roads, in a deserted barn we sneaked into, in fields of wildflowers, and sometimes in the backseat of her car if we couldn't wait to get back to the apartment. I think she came into my life to encourage me to loosen up and to have fun, and to be a kid again. *(Claire, 66)*

For about a decade, on and off, I had an ongoing, casual sexual relationship with a next-door neighbor, a handsome, vigorous man with a strong sex drive who was happy to indulge me any time I asked. I liked this arrangement— being able to ask for sex when I wanted it. His body was model perfect: gorgeous, lean, muscled, and sleek as a panther, with skin so smooth and a scent so sweet that I loved to rub my face up and down his chest and belly. I would phone or call out to his yard to invite him to come over, and we would tumble into bed on the spot. Once, I called him and said, "I've got something that needs fixing. Is there a handyman in the house?" He came over wearing nothing but a tool belt and an erection. *(Kassie, 62)*

Right after my first divorce, when I was twenty-three, I was hanging out at a lounge, my stomping grounds, dancing with a man I had talked with a few times before. He was a thin, homely man, not my type at all, but he had a fantastic personality. He looked me in the eye and whispered, "I don't have a very big penis, but I can lick my eyebrows." I busted out laughing, but he said, "I dare you to find out." I thought about how much fun he was and how bad I was for judging someone because he wasn't a Greek god. We went home together, and I spent three days and nights in bed with this man. He was a sexual dynamo and taught me things I had never even heard of before. He was magnificent, and after that, I never again judged a book by its cover. He was married, and I was dating someone else at the time—it was a one-time fling for us both. *(Catherine, 65)*

After nine months of crazy-making celibacy when I was in my fifties, a good friend—a gay man who was in a stable, long-term relationship—approached me. He was frustrated because he wanted sex more frequently than his partner did. He was afraid that an affair with another man might threaten his primary relationship and be risky healthwise. He knew I really missed sex. Although he liked me a lot, he knew that sex with a woman would always take second place to sex with a man, so his relationship with his life partner was in no danger from me. After discussion and setting ground rules, his partner agreed to our sleeping together. My friend and I started meeting once a week for sex and companionship. It was comfortable and affectionate, and it took the edge off our raging libidos. This continued for two years, until I fell in love with the man I wanted to be with exclusively. We're close, platonic friends now, and we laugh that we kept each other out of trouble. *(Diana, 62)*

Coupled and Free

Richard was married when I first met him. He was handsome, charismatic, brilliant, and troubled, and I was attracted to him immediately. He told me that he and his wife had an "understanding," and I talked myself into believing him. We had a marvelous time talking about literature, but when we switched from book talk to pillow talk, it was only so-so. We went back to books.

We met again after Richard was divorced, and the sparks flew, igniting a forest fire that hurled us into a passionate affair and an unexpected emotional connection. We became a couple but insisted that we would continue to "see" other people. We were having wonderful sex, but we were both hooked on variety and the exhilaration of a liberated life.

At the time, I had two other sex buddies (one from the "twelve lively women" ad, the other a long-term friend) whom I met with occasionally. While I wanted to be with Richard primarily, I still wanted my freedom. Richard was a sexual huntsman, turned on by attraction and seduction, and was thrilled with an agreement that allowed him a combination of freedom and connection. We agreed to be honest with each other and found ourselves turned on by hearing the other's stories.

Then, a dear friend who had been a past lover discovered that he was HIV positive. He told me, and I took the ELISA (Enzyme Linked Immuno-Sorbent Assay) HIV antibody test—it was positive.

I can barely express how my world flipped upside down in an instant.

The counselor told me that the ELISA test sometimes gave false positives. I would need to have the Western Blot test, which was more accurate. The time between getting this news and the Western Blot results was the longest two weeks of my life.

The results of the second test: negative.

Richard and I took this scare as a warning to look really closely at how dangerously we were living. We decided to give up our wild ways and settle into monogamous couplehood. At least, that was the agreement. I learned after we broke up that Richard resumed having sex with other women at some point and neglected to tell me about it. He never knew that I found out. Perhaps he's learning it now, reading this book.

Love and Commitment

When I fell in love with Robert and we committed to each other exclusively, I knew beyond any doubt that I could promise fidelity. Robert was uneasy about getting involved with me at first because his background was much more traditional—he had had some youthful explorations, a long, faithful marriage, and a few steady relationships after his divorce. When I met him, he had been celibate for four years, and I was having a sex-buddy relationship with a male friend.

Robert had no desire to participate in my kind of lifestyle and made it clear from the beginning that exclusivity was an absolute requirement if we were to get involved. He was concerned that I would be unhappy, unwilling, or restless in a committed relationship.

I had a dream that I visited men of my past, told them about my relationship with Robert, and then had "farewell sex" with each of them before leaving. When I told Robert my dream, he was worried that eventually I would desire other men and have a

Sexually Seasoned Women Speak about Settling Down

I was blessed to be in my twenties during the PPPA period: Post-Pill Pre-AIDS. I was looking for love in the wrong places—mainly bars. Of course, I found plenty of willing sex partners, but not many particularly interesting men looking for a relationship. I regret not developing and following my own interests and meeting men in that way. I would have found more stable and interesting men if I had. I would never look for a partner in a bar now. *(Melanie, 64)*

I now know how nice, secure, and important it is to have sex with one partner, the right one. I'm way more traditional now. *(Joanna, 61)*

Now I have a very satisfactory partner relationship, and it's based more on companionship, love, and fun than on lust. I've lived with the same man for about seven years now. We have a committed relationship, although we have discussed that there is always the possibility of a passing sexual encounter, perhaps when traveling. I think if that happened, we wouldn't mention it. *(Phoebe, 64)*

At about age forty-eight, I was dating and sexually active with three wonderful women. It was so exciting! I was honest about my sex relationships with all of them. After about six months, one of them said she wanted to be in a monogamous relationship and I would have to decide. I really did love her, so it was not too difficult to say goodbye to the other two women. I was beyond the flirting stage and ready to settle down. *(Kendall, 69)*

I've been married for twenty-three years. Originally it was an open relationship, and he still has a long-term friendship that was once sexual with a woman friend, but there hasn't been much outside activity for a number of years. We're too busy and not as inclined as we once were. I've calmed down a lot. *(Tina, 61)*

I used to be hooked on variety. I had trouble sustaining sexual interest in a long-term relationship. I often felt my interest waning after six months, and if I got past a year, I had to kick up my fantasy life several notches to stay aroused with my partner. But now, I feel very different, and I'm so in love that I cannot imagine my attention wandering, much less my body parts. I don't know how much is hormones settling down and how much is having found the perfect man finally. I have no doubt that I'm here to stay. *(Diana, 62)*

difficult time staying true to my commitment, or that I'd go off with someone else in spite of that commitment.

But no, I know what my dream meant: I was truly ready to give up that part of my life. I was saying goodbye in my dream the way I had said hello to this new life, and now that part was over.

I had no doubt then, and my commitment remains as strong as a bond can be. I've tried everything I've wanted to try, and I've done enough experimenting for a lifetime. I know this absolutely. Robert offers me far more than great sex—he offers me the love of a lifetime.

CHAPTER 13

Late Bloomers— Ready to Fly

Life is either a daring adventure or nothing at all. Security is mostly a superstition. It does not exist in nature.

—Helen Keller

As you read in the last chapter, many of the women I interviewed had sowed their wild oats as young women and were now settled comfortably into satisfying, monogamous relationships. But if you think that's the only way to ease into the last third of life,

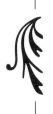

> *If I had my life to live again, I'd make the same mistakes, only sooner.*
> —Tallulah Bankhead

think again! I heard from plenty of women who were not camp followers of the sexual revolution. Some married early, some came of age long before the sixties, and some broke loose sexually later—often after a divorce or widowhood, sometimes in an arrangement with a long-term partner.

Many of these women report that they're enjoying the wildest, most satisfying sex of their lives right now!

Bea's Story: Discovering Passion with a Young Lover

Bea, seventy-seven, is enjoying a vibrant sexual relationship with a much younger man. Here is her story in her own words:

I love sex, and I look forward to it. I have a lover thirty years younger. I met him twelve years ago. He was doing some remodeling for my mother. We stared at each other, and my mother yelled, "She's sixty-five!" He got up and left.

Several years later, I hired him to do my remodeling. He made all the moves. He began by touching me casually, touching my shoulder or hand and not letting go. He would rub my arm or touch my breast. Pretty soon, we were going at it.

My husband was still alive when I started the affair, but it had been ten full years since I'd had sex. My husband had diabetes and couldn't do it, and he wouldn't go to a doctor about it. Sex was different with my lover—he was much more skillful and open than my husband.

I consider myself very lustful. I have frequent orgasms, and I climax very easily because he's large and skillful. Orgasms are easier using intercourse, fingers, tongues, and vibrators. My lover uses dildos on me. He brings porno-graphic movies and other things to help teach me. I said, "Did you bring those so I would learn what to do?" He said, "Yes." He has taken the lead in all these areas. Now I can't stop him, and I don't want to.

My lover talks about getting married. I say, "Oh, no way." I've been married three times before. Women change once they marry.

I told my family I had a boyfriend, and the reactions were very negative. My son-in-law said, "You should see a psychiatrist." Now he realizes how happy I am.

This is the happiest time of my life. I'm enjoying my old age more than any other time. I'm financially indepen-dent, and I can do whatever I want all day long. In 1998, I had a stroke, and I thought I would die. But instead, I'm going full steam ahead in every way. I never expected to be so happy at this age.

When One Night Will Do: Sex with the Imperfect Stranger

In my active dating days, I thrust out my chin and proclaimed that I'd rather regret something I did than something I didn't do. So I took risks, plenty of them. I'm very lucky that I never contracted a sexually transmitted disease in the days before we got careful about condoms, and I never was physically hurt or worse by partners I barely knew.

When I was younger, my sex fantasies often revolved around perfect strangers: men (young and sweet, wearing long, curly hair and nothing else) who were so entranced by me that all they wanted to do was pleasure me. In my carefree thirties, I would occasionally (okay, rarely) meet the almost-perfect stranger, flirt with my heart pounding, and, once in a great while (okay, three times total), have a one-night stand.

Unfortunately, the fantasy was always a million times better than the reality. The stranger was, after all, someone who got off on sex with a stranger, and "got off" was the operative term. If I got anything out of it, it was frustration and knowing that I had made a huge mistake. One of them just wanted to masturbate in front of me. Another helped me through what otherwise would have been a lonely birthday, and didn't mind the menstrual blood that stained the hotel room sheets, but never answered my phone calls when I tried to see him again. The third—I hate to admit it, but I remember nothing about him.

I know that many women, young and older, do enjoy sex with strangers. Others wouldn't put this at the top of their to-do lists, but if there's no steady lover, no good friend who wants to be a sex buddy, and no dashing date in sight, hey, it's a step above another Saturday night with Ben & Jerry.

Women who have been out of the dating game for a long time and are hungry to cool their sexual jets with a partner sometimes throw out caution with their inhibitions. If sex with a stranger is your thing, I'm not moralizing—I'm just urging you to be more careful than I was. Know the person's name and phone number, and something about him or her. Use safe sex barriers—do not believe anything a horny date tells you about HIV or STD status. Let a friend know what you're doing, with whom, and when and where. Promise to phone the next day to let your friend know you're okay. Worst-case scenario, someone will know to bang on your door if you don't call. Best case, you can laugh about it.

Jaime's Story: Upbringing vs. Desire

Jaime, seventy-three, is a beautiful, lively woman who's youthful in appearance, energy, and spirit, and who still battles guilt from a strict upbringing and a long, unhappy marriage. Here she talks about her experiences and feelings:

> *I was only with my husband, except for one slight indiscretion, and then we got a divorce. We reconciled and spent another thirty years together. I was miserable with my husband. The "indiscretion" was with a really good friend. He was cute—pants pressed, shoes shined, and really nice to talk to. It happened two or three times. I was madly in love with this man, and I dreamed about him leaving his wife.*
>
> *At fifty-one, I was divorced and alone for the first time in my life. It was an emotional time for me, and I was a wreck for a while. I had sex with someone who talked dirty talk the whole time—that was really different for me. We dated for a year or more. He wanted to turn on the light, and I said, "No way!" I'm a very inhibited person. I never want anybody seeing me without my clothes on!*
>
> *I met this guy, twenty years younger, whom I had seen*

a few times at a dance. He came to do some repair work. He offered to give me a massage. One thing led to another, and he spent the night. I didn't have enough self-esteem to say no. I was raised to think you do what other people want you to do. I was so depressed after that. It was not a relationship. He also took me for about $300—he promised to pay me back. It was really awful.

An old boyfriend called me—we had stayed friends for years. I went over to his house after not seeing him for a while, and I ended up naked dancing with him. We made love on the floor. I am very inhibited, so I don't know how that happened. I still blush about that, and it was ten years ago.

I have experimented a little more with some partners. One man has been a friend and lover off and on for years. He notices when I get new earrings or new shoes. We've had oral sex, which seems more intimate than intercourse. I never thought I would, but I really enjoyed doing it to him. I won't have intercourse with him. Every time he gets near me with his fingers, I get really excited. But I don't want to let him touch me there and not reciprocate by letting him inside of me—it's not fair, even though he says it's okay.

Leona and Bob: Loving Their Friends

Leona, seventy-seven, and Bob, seventy-six, have been together for sixty years. They were high school sweethearts who married young, and they still enjoy a strong relationship, including an active sex life. "Sex makes me happy," says Leona. "I'm very simplistic—it just makes me happy."

I first met Leona and Bob in 1970. My husband (at the time) and I moved in across the street from them and became observers of their whirlwind world. Two of the most loving and generous people I've ever met, they shared freely of their time, knowledge, and home. So many children went in and out of their house that it was six months before I could be sure which ones were their own children, which were their children's friends, who preferred being in such a joyful home, and which were children whom Leona and Bob had taken in and were parenting, short-term or long-term. They were terrific people, exceptional parents, a devoted couple, and, in their leisure time, foot soldiers of the sexual revolution. Leona and Bob enjoyed having sex with close friends—and they still do.

"We were monogamous—if you define it as not having intercourse with other people—for the first twenty years," Bob explains. "But if you define monogamous as not having an interest in anyone else, then never."

During the sixties, Bob said to Leona, "I feel like you might like to have sex with other men." She replied, "Yes, I would." He said he felt the same way.

"My wife was the first to have sexual relations with a good friend of the family, and it didn't bother me," says Bob. "To me, that was her decision. It did not affect our intimacy." Shortly after that, Bob started having his own outside relationships. "I never felt guilty unless I didn't let my wife know I wouldn't be home when she expected me," he says.

"It was during the make-love-not-war time, and we were all defiant rabble-rousers," says Leona. "It used to be that I'd get involved with someone because we were friends, or

Late Bloomers Speak about Early Relationships

I had a very blah sex life my entire marriage, for eighteen years. I thought there was something wrong with me because I totally shut myself down sexually. We had sex from time to time, but it was passionless. It was a bad marriage—I was angry with my husband, and he was angry with me. He eventually left me for a younger woman. *(Erica, 62)*

I was monogamous when I was married—except for one fling after my second husband came home and told me he had a venereal disease. After I was cured, I had a one-nighter with the friend of a friend. *(Kaycee, 66)*

In my first marriage, I married someone who was a sexual mismatch for me. He was afraid of sex, came from a restrictive Catholic background, and had premature orgasms. I believed in the "save yourself for marriage" philosophy at that time, but if I had had sex prior to marriage with this man, I wouldn't have married him. This lack of sex in my first marriage catapulted me into marrying the

for camaraderie, or because we were camping—any excuse. It wasn't just a feel-good thing. We wanted to embrace our friends."

"Our relationships evolved through long-term friendships," echoes Bob. "I enjoy sex with close friends—it's a way of expressing that I enjoy the other person."

Now that the couple is older, they have fewer outside rela-

second time because of great sex, but again he wasn't a good match for me. So sex—or the lack of sex—took me down two wrong paths. *(Lily, 60)*

My first relationship was a fourteen-year monogamous relationship. We never made love in the light, always in the dark. It was exciting at first because we were new to it and enthralled by each other. We felt safe—it's you and me against the world. But as it went along, I wanted to experiment more, but I felt ashamed of wanting that, and my partner didn't have any sexual curiosity. She was a pretty strict Catholic. It eventually got pretty boring. I left that relationship, started meeting lesbians who were active, read books like *The Joy of Lesbian Sex*, and experimented more sexually. *(Claire, 66)*

I wish my husband or my former lover had been as joyful and playful as my most recent lover. If my husband had done some of the things that this lover did, we might still be together. There was too much seriousness with my husband, and too much reluctance with my former lover. *(Rachel, 62)*

tionships, but their belief system hasn't changed much. "Sex is fun—I really like it," says Bob. "But it's always combined with a relationship. Some women I've had sexual relationships with in the past, but sex isn't part of the relationship anymore. I'm still close with all these women. Now, I have some sexual relationships that mean a great deal to me. With some, we might have sex just every couple of years, depending on circumstances,

Stories Your Grandmother Didn't Tell You: Late Bloomers Speak about Busting Loose

It had been ten years since I was sexually active, and frankly, I thought I was finished with it all. I joined a gym to get my poor, pathetic body into something resembling a woman. Then, post-menopausal zest hit me with a huge wave of pure lust. I had this overwhelming urge to jump my trainer! I was sitting at his feet, and he was wearing those cute little baggy shorts. I almost put my hand up his pants. At first I thought I could handle it, but I couldn't think about anything else. So I told him I wanted to sleep with him, and he was very charming about it. He told me I had balls to tell him, but nothing happened. I ultimately transferred to another gym. I then decided that I needed to get back in action. Right now, I am having the time of my life. Since I only have so much time left, I'm going for the gold! *(Kaycee, 66)*

After I separated from my husband, I really came alive. Basically, I thought I'd never be interested in sex again. But I was interested in sex, just not with my husband. Nine months after we separated, at age sixty, I went nuts. I started becoming ravenous about men again, as I had been in my thirties. This was a great surprise to me. I really thought it was over. All this desire came flooding back— pent-up demand after all those years of no sexual satisfaction. I had been very sexual in my thirties, and this was just as good, sometimes better. I got turned on easily, and I had orgasms easily. It was quite a revelation. *(Erica, 62)*

I've been alone for twelve years, and I've been through a lot, and I think I'm awake finally. I spent fifty years of my life not knowing if I had a right to what I felt, shamed by my sexual feelings. I was in therapy for fifteen years and did major work. Now, I can feel sexual when and where I want to. I feel better about myself than I ever expected—freer to be myself, to go to those places I was reluctant to go before, and willing to share my fantasies with a partner and to make love in those ways I always fantasized about but never had the courage to do before. *(Claire, 66)*

I was fifty-eight, and he was forty. It was the most amazing sexual experience I'd ever had. This man really liked the acts of sexual intimacy. We were not in love, and we didn't want anything from each other except the joy of the moment. I'd had several orgasms and was, frankly, getting tired physically, although I was still engaged in the wonder of it all when he paused and said, "I don't know why I'm so out of breath—we haven't been doing it for very long." We'd been "doing it" for half an hour or so, and I thought, "Wow. This is great. He doesn't think this has gone on very long." I'd had lovers who would go down on me but never a lover who regarded it as one of the many joys of sex. This man was skilled and inventive. He might've been scribing the alphabet with his tongue; it was divine. *(Rachel, 62)*

and other relationships are more consistent and long-term, over twenty years. Some of my partners are very close friends with my wife; others don't interest her as friends."

"My philosophy hasn't changed much over the decades," says Leona. "However, my personal life has changed because now I'm only involved with one other person besides my husband, and it's a long-term relationship. I'm not sure in this day and age if I'd go about it the same way. Today is a different time and a different way of looking at things. I'm happy that my kids appear to be monogamous and very happy."

≈ CHAPTER 14

Sparking the Familiar Fire: How to Spice Up a Long-Term Relationship

Love doesn't just sit there like a stone; it has to be made, like bread, remade all the time, made new.
                    —Ursula K. LeGuin in *The Lathe of Heaven*

The blaze of lust that ignites and consumes us when we're new to each other does settle down after years in a relationship. But that doesn't mean that the sizzle has to fizzle. We can use our creativity to devise spicy activities and fantasies that keep the home fires burning.

Since Robert and I need a long stretch of time for our love-making, we make a point of scheduling quality time together, no matter how busy we are. Our relationship is a high priority. We know we can't skip watering the garden and still expect the flowers to thrive. Likewise, we can't just plant daisies and expect the blooms to take our breath away. Being in an exclusive relationship offers us the opportunity to find creative ways to spice up our sex life and keep it new and surprising.

I know that four years together does not make me a specialist in long-term relationships, and I'd be a laughingstock if I claimed to have all the solutions for keeping the spark going after decades—I've never done it. So, I consulted my interviewees who know the secrets to relationship longevity and walk their talk. Here are some stories from satisfied women in loving, decades-long relationships, describing how they keep the sparks flying:

Tana, Age Sixty, On Her Forty-Year Relationship

I was a child bride—or so I tell everyone—who was still in college when I said "I do." The best thing about sex at my age is the feeling of closeness with my husband. It's easier to face aging and body changes that reduce sexual feelings and performance when you are comfortable and relaxed with your partner.

I've always worn the same perfume, from adolescence to the present. My husband loves it and identifies it as how I smell. He often hugs me and buries his face in my neck, saying, "You smell nice!" That always makes me feel desirable, which is a turn-on.

Even if you don't feel like it, accept any advance your partner makes, unless you have a very good reason to reject it. Men our age aren't always able to perform as well as they used to, and they're very sensitive to rejection. If they don't "use it," they lose it even faster than we women do. So, if your man is ready, don't miss the opportunity—the sex is likely to be much better than at times when he's not feeling so ready. And with success after success, you'll find that your partner—and you—will be ready, successful, and fulfilled much more often. More really is better!

The more we continue to have frequent sex, the better the chances we'll both have a great time. One really effective thing I do is apply a small amount of K-Y Jelly every night before bed—it's very effective as a moisturizer, but that's not its most important effect. It eases initial entry, so then my natural moisture can take over. And since it's a regular routine, I'm always "ready."

But it's not what you do in bed that's most important; it's what you do every day to keep your shared sensual life active. If your partner has lost the habit of spontaneous kisses and hugs, now's the time to start asking, "Do you have a minute? I need a hug!" If your partner is sitting watching television, put your arms around him, or lie down and put your head in his lap. If you're taking a walk, hold hands. That feeling of closeness during the day can really rev you up for more action at night.

If you have an affectionate dog or cat, it's obvious to you that this approach works. You come home, and the dog runs to

---

Sexually Seasoned Women Share Spicy Tidbits

We've been together for sixteen years in a committed, exclusive relationship. My husband does amazing things with his tongue. I think he could raise me from a coma. *(Susie, 60)*

One of my favorite things is smoothing chocolate mousse onto his penis and licking it off very slowly. If there's anything better than chocolate, it's my lover's chocolate-covered penis. Yum. *(Diana, 62)*

When I know he's watching around bedtime, I undress very slowly, doing other things in between. I go bra-less out to dinner and grab his butt discreetly in public. I say things like, "How is my sexy guy today?" I shave the back of his neck for him and then nibble on his ears. I rub his

---

the door, jumping up and down, wagging his tail, licking your hands, nuzzling your legs. You know you are loved and desired, and that makes you love your pet even more and enjoy those moments of snuggling, petting, and scratching his tummy.

Mary Ann, Age Sixty-two, On Her Forty-Three-Year Relationship

Keeping a long-term sexual relationship fulfilling takes a commitment to looking for and trying new things, whether it's sex toys, movies, books, new locations for sex, or otherwise changing the routine. Exploring each other's bodies (and minds) to find new ways of pleasing each other

inner thighs after giving him a neck rub. I like it when he holds me gently and for a long time, nibbling on my toes, caressing my legs and buttocks, and "eating" his way up my legs. We've been in a committed, exclusive relationship for twenty-three years. *(Ulla, 61)*

I love when he rubs on me a strawberry-smelling scent that we found in a women's sex shop—it makes me feel like I'm in a field of strawberries. *(Pepper, 71)*

We like it wild. We like innocent bondage with silk ties, but nothing that isn't honoring each other. We can be as wild and outrageous as we want, or we can be calm and quiet, just touching. There are no expectations, and no feeling that there might be failure. Whatever we end up doing is wonderful. I love the sense of being close and warm and open with a partner. *(Monica, 60)*

is ongoing—after forty-three years of marriage, we're still discovering new things.

My husband and I are enjoying a better sexual and personal relationship than ever. Our relationship is and always has been monogamous. With commitment to each other and a willingness to explore, sex stays exciting and fun and has enriched our relationship tremendously.

We're both busy with outside commitments, so we schedule two or three evenings a week together and are always looking for new ways to get and give pleasure. We look forward to our evenings and don't feel in any way that planning sex is unromantic.

I like to initiate a snuggle or some low-key sex play or teasing as a warm-up to sex. The teasing consists of long, sensual hugs, some back rubbing for me, enough playing with nipples (direct) and genitals (through clothes) to keep the arousal level ratcheted up, and some talk about what each of us plans to do to the other when we have an evening together again. Sometimes it involves some fellatio, which I find more arousing than just about anything else. Generally speaking, during the day, we see each other only at mealtime and during the evening, so there is time apart between these encounters.

Although I've always liked and wanted sex, it took a long time (and much help from a great husband) to overcome a lot of hang-ups about sex. Early on, I was not willing to try oral sex, sex toys, erotic movies or books, bondage, or anything much but the missionary position in our bedroom. We've gotten more relaxed and adventuresome as we've aged, and we have sought out instructional books and soft-core videos. There are newer ones (many produced and/or directed by women) geared to couples that are well done as well as arousing to watch.

We use sex toys routinely. We like a couple of vibrators— a hand-held flat one and a penis-shaped one—and furs and feathers.

Essential to me is the trust built from my husband's desire to give me pleasure. We have learned what the other likes and find giving the other pleasure the best aphrodisiac. Any performance anxiety went away years ago. Talking with each other about sexual wishes and seeking out new sex aids and new approaches has worked for us. We continue to find new ways to orally or manually stimulate each other—just putting pressure on a new spot or changing a movement can bring new sensations.

We've also explored mild bondage. I tie my husband's legs and arms to the corners of our bed or in a spread-out position standing up, and I tease him for a long time, ending with either backing up onto his penis (the first time I did this he very nearly went crazy) or giving him a blowjob. Oral sex for me comes either before or after, but the bondage is the turn-on. Our bondage equipment consists of hooks on our bed frame and a closet door and dog collars with sheepskin on the skin side.

My husband also recently discovered a device called Aneros (www.malegspot.com), which extends the period he can go before ejaculating. It allows us to enjoy each other longer and allows me to give him what I can only call multiple orgasms, by hand and mouth, without an ejaculation. I find this extremely arousing! This device has a small "finger" that is inserted anally and presses on his prostate, with another finger-like part that puts gentle pressure on his perineum. It has extended our lovemaking sessions, and—what I like best—when we finish without an ejaculation, it leaves him in a snuggly and romantic mood for a few days, until the next time. We recently tried Viagra, which I thought was unnecessary considering my husband's normal stamina, but it does extend the time he can stay erect, which is nice.

Fatigue, preoccupation with outside concerns, and stubborn inhibitions still derail us occasionally. We don't consider it significant—there will be another opportunity soon.

Sexually Seasoned Women Speak about How They Spice Up a Long-Term Relationship

On our first anniversary, we traveled across the United States by train. We are about to leave for a romantic replay, this time taking the cross-Canada train—and at a much more luxurious level than our first trip! On that first trip, he spent lots of time reading to me—he's great at reading aloud—and we're already talking about which book to choose for this trip. In my opinion, there's nothing more romantic than being closed up in a little compartment, sitting face-to-face as beautiful scenery passes by, daytime and nighttime. *(Gerri, 60)*

Having the same loving partner for twenty-three years has its benefits. We are totally relaxed, and there's no nervousness about pleasing each other, no pressure, no issues. Our lovemaking is not goal-oriented, it's process-oriented. Orgasms are a bonus, not the goal. Neither of us is in the same shape we were even five years ago, but our relationship is so loving and giving that it doesn't matter. I can tell him whatever is in my mind, and he'll listen and respond thoughtfully. We laugh a lot and make silly jokes during sex. That, plus our intimate physical knowledge of each other, is as good as it gets for me. Spicing it up is not important to me. We have a blend of sexuality, sensuality, spirituality, love, and closeness that just can't be beat. *(Tina, 61)*

We talk! We have sweet words that mean something special for both of us. We find new and different activities, and we're willing to adventure into these new arenas together. We travel together, preferably to places neither of us has been before—and certainly not with a previous partner! We write love notes and leave them around the house, in the car, or in each other's pockets, where we'll be surprised to find them. We plan surprise dates at least once a month to some romantic place or event. We try new things, especially in our sex life! We laugh often with—but never at— each other. *(Kendall, 69)*

At bedtime, I occasionally wear something really sexy, like just a lace shawl. I'll make suggestive remarks early in the evening to let him know that I'd rather he didn't stay working on the computer until late. We have little weekend getaways to romantic inns. I am married to a wonderful man who is eleven years younger than I, and we regularly have sex. *(Susie, 60)*

I try to be honest about sex and talk openly. I read studies and share this info with my partner to get rid of the myths and misinformation. I feel lucky that I always have had orgasms because sex was considered natural and was discussed openly in my family. I feel that my partner and I meet most of each other's needs and expectations because of this openness. *(Lily, 60)*

My lover doesn't seem to need spicing. What turns me on is just him, the whole of him—who he is, what he looks like, how he treats me, and more. We've been together thirty years, starting out as an open relationship (mostly for him) and then becoming exclusive and committed after about four years. *(Pepper, 71)*

Penny, Age Sixty, On Her Thirty-Eight-Year Relationship

For my husband's birthday, I shaved my yoni and did a very sexy dance in a teddy while he lay on the bed, and he loved it.

When I look back over all the years we have been together and all that has occurred in our lives, I appreciate my husband so much. Over the years, we have worked together in different businesses, raised great kids, now have two grandkids with another on the way, and have shared so much. He is a fantastic father and a supportive partner who adores me. We still find each other attractive and turn each other on.

My husband and I go out of our way to do nice things for each other and to say sweet things. We like to have date nights, when we go out to dinner or the movies. He makes me laugh, and we have a good time together. Being silly and just having fun together is so important.

He has always been interested in sex, even when I wasn't, but he didn't make me feel guilty about it. My husband is much more unconditionally loving than I am, but I have other qualities that complement the relationship. What I'm trying to say is that because of all that we've been through together, it makes the intimacy during sex much sweeter.

I am very grateful to feel so alive, sexy, and in love with my husband after so many years together.

Kindling for the Fire

"I got something in the mail I want to use with you," I tell Robert on the phone.

Tenderness and Titillation

Dell Williams, eighty-two, founder of Eve's Garden, shares suggestions for romantic and sensual preludes to lovemaking:

How about a little foreplay in the form of relief from the stresses of modern life, a splendid meal in a quiet atmosphere, a long soak in scented bathwater, or a tender and intimate full-body massage? How about a revival of courtship rituals in relationships, an environment of flowers, and music, and candles? How about setting aside some prime time for sex? . . . I suggest reading or viewing erotica together as a prelude to sex play; cuddling to enhance mutual relaxation and affection; masturbation to climax prior to penetration to provide both ample arousal and a guarantee of satisfaction; exploration of techniques and positions and sex toys new to the partners to provide a sense of adventure and excitement in what might have become the exercise of routine duty.

—from *Revolution in the Garden:*
Memoirs of the Gardenkeeper,[1]
by Dell Williams and Lynn Vannucci

"Oh?" he says, making the word rise and fall into several syllables. "The last time you got something in the mail, it was pretty good." Over the phone line, we picture each other smiling at recent memories of our favorite purchases.

Keeping a Long-Term Relationship Fresh and Sexually Hot

Here are some tips from couples' therapist Tina B. Tessina, PhD:

Romance has been blown out of proportion in our culture. It is a momentary, fleeting thing, and it does add excitement to your relationship, but it's not a way of life. You can't keep it going every moment through the stress and business of everyday life. However, it is a very useful tool to reassure each other that you are still in love. Whenever there's a lack of romance or excitement between you, recharge your connection and celebrate your mutual love, affection, and desire with these events and rituals:

• Arrange a date, a present, a surprise, a joke, or a hug when your partner needs a boost.

• Meet at a singles bar and pretend to pick each other up.

• Take a special vacation to a romantic spot together.

• One evening a week, have a "date," and do things you did when you first met.

• Have breakfast in bed or a romantic picnic in the park.

• Send a card, a plant, flowers, cologne, or another present for no special occasion.

• Take a class together in something you'll enjoy (mountain climbing, dancing, skiing, acting, rollerblading, pottery making, painting, stained glass, sailing, swimming, cooking), or get involved in your community to create new experiences together.

When your relationship lasts for a while, your lovemaking will change. As you get closer, passion no longer grows automatically out of the excitement of the new and unknown.

Rather than allowing your energy to subside, you can allow your lovemaking to change and grow, deepening as your partnership does. Couples who develop a "sexual repertoire" that includes a variety of sexual habits, attitudes, and options report feeling more satisfaction and freedom to express their love with enough variety that they never get bored. These suggestions will help you create a variety of experiences together.

Quickies let you have sex when you don't really have time for a full, leisurely, romantic evening. One of you can give oral sex before you leave for work, pet the other to climax in the car at a drive-in movie, use vibrators together to have orgasms without a lot of foreplay late at night, or take a nap and then have a "quickie" before rushing off to a party.

Sneaky Sex has the added excitement of "forbidden fruit": having silent sex behind locked doors while there are guests in your home, sneaking lovemaking in any place that reminds you of your childhood, visiting your partner at work, and having quickie sex on the couch in a locked office.

Romantic Sex is the full-blown variety: candlelight, dinner, quiet talking, dressing up, and perhaps a lovely hotel room or a romantic dinner for two when you have time alone at home. Romantic sex is especially good for anniversaries, Valentine's Day, or anytime your relationship needs a boost.

New Couple Sex allows you to recreate a scene from your dating days as closely as possible: the time you met at church and couldn't wait to get home and make love, the flowers you used to bring home as a surprise, or saying all the silly, wildly-in-love things you said then.

continued on next page

continued from page 217

Making-Up Sex happens after you've had an argument or a struggle and forgiven each other; lovemaking can be extra tender and memorable.

Comforting Sex is wonderful when one of you is sad or stressed and the other is especially caring and soothing, doing all of your favorite things to comfort and relax you.

Relaxing Sex is the kind to do on a weekend morning, when you have no obligations and can laze around, have breakfast in bed, and make love for as long as you want. There's no pressure, no hurry, and no demands on each other.

Reassuring Sex is affection and intimacy intended to reassure a partner who is temporarily insecure, or to reaffirm your mutual love and commitment to each other. It is often accompanied by many verbal declarations of love and explaining again why you are so important to each other.

"Don't tell me what it is," he requests. "Surprise me."

The surprise is the Kama Sutra Bedside Box, an antique-looking, painted wooden box containing small containers of Honey Dust (in a satin pouch, with a feather applicator), skin-warming Oil of Love, Love Liquid lubricant, and Vanilla Crème Massage Cream. All but the lubricant are edible. A sensual guide promises great delights with these "tools of the trade" for lovemaking, all of which are available from www.kamasutra.com. Many of us remember Kama Sutra oils, lotions, and powders from the sexual heydays of the sixties; it's the same company and with the same focus. It will be fun to return to the

Fantasy Sex allows you to act out all the silly, forbidden, or exciting fantasies: nurse and patient, two children "playing house," master or dominatrix and slave, stripper and customer, extraterrestrial alien and abductee, famous movie star and adoring fan, your two favorite characters from a soap opera, novel, or movie, or anything else you can imagine. This is a great time for costumes, masks, sexual toys, leather outfits, or whatever enhancements you enjoy.

The possible varieties of sexual attitudes, environments, energies, and activities are truly endless. No matter how exciting any of the above options seems at first, if it is all you do, it will become boring eventually—and no matter how tame the option is, if you haven't done it for a while, it will refresh and revitalize your experience of each other.[2]

Tina B. Tessina, PhD, is a psychologist and author of How to Be a Couple and Still Be Free *(www.tinatessina.com).*

familiar sweet-and-spicy scents we remember from our younger days, thirty years later.

As much as we continue to find each other new and exciting, and often making love has all the magic of discovering each other for the first time, we acknowledge the importance of bringing something new and unexpected into our bed. I used to crave variety in relationships, which I acted on by going to a new lover whenever I felt the thrill was gone and predictability had settled in. Now there's no danger of that—our relationship is solid and exhilarating and full of creativity. Variety takes place in our interactions with each other.

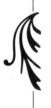

A good marriage is one which allows for change and growth in the individuals and in the way they express their love.

—Pearl Buck

The well-known psychotherapist Lawrence LeShan, whom I have the great pleasure of knowing as Uncle Larry, had a dynamic fifty-eight-year marriage with parent educator and author Eda LeShan until her death in 2002. He tells me that surprising each other is essential to keeping love vibrant. In any relationship, he says, once it gets to pure ritual—what we say and do are predictable, almost scripted—we stop noticing each other. We already know what's going to happen. "Surprise each other," he suggests. "Bring a single flower, wear something unexpected, do something completely original and different, reach out for each other in a new way."

Although Robert used to scoff at my propensity for buying sex toys, new lubricants, books, and other boudoir accoutrements over the Internet and at local erotic shops, now he's open to just about any new experience I come up with. We've discovered some marvelous playthings and helpmates that enhance our lovemaking and keep it fresh. We've also accumulated enough unwanted accessories for a garage sale—videos and books we personally don't find sexy, toys that make us laugh instead of moan, lubricants that are too thick or thin or dry too fast—let me know if you want to arrange a "sassy women swap session"!

CHAPTER 15

When You or Your Partner Can't

We don't see things as they are. We see them as we are.
—Anaïs Nin

I started out thinking this chapter—originally titled "When Your Partner Can't or Doesn't"—would be about how women cope in relationships with men who experience erectile dysfunction. According to the spam I receive in my email box daily, ED is *the* major concern of men—and an advertiser's dream. I am reminded of this joke that a male friend used to tell me:

Question: What's the difference between fear and panic?

Answer: Fear is the first time you can't get it up twice. Panic is the second time you can't get it up once.

According to a 1994 study, 67 percent of the men surveyed at age seventy experienced mild-to-severe ED. A partner's ED is an important challenge for some of the women I interviewed, and I am grateful for their candor about this intimate part of their lives. You'll read some of their comments here. Many have found that sex can be satisfying when both partners communicate and seek creative and loving solutions, whatever the penis is or is not able to do.

Erectile dysfunction, not to minimize its importance, is only part of the big picture, though. The sexual challenges of aging bodies go beyond penis problems.

The fact is that *both* partners may have health problems to deal with that affect sex. Arthritis, osteoporosis, heart disease, cancer—all of these impact our sex lives as well as our daily living. These and many other health problems require relationship adjustments, including an extra dose of understanding from our partners. While health problems are certainly not the exclusive domain of genarians in the upper ranges, they occur with more frequency in older adults.

It's ironic, isn't it? We're at the prime time of life to enjoy sex. We know ourselves and our partners, the kids are long gone, we have more leisure time, we're less driven, and our partners have learned how to satisfy us. What a cruel twist of fate that this is the time our bodies start acting up with aches, pains, and chronic diseases!

Faced with problems from bad knees and back pain to life-threatening illnesses, partners become collaborators, discovering creative solutions in the name of love. We explore new positions and props, such as wedge-shaped pillows that lift, tilt, and support (our favorite: the Ramp, available from www.blowfish.com/catalog/toys/cushions.html). We take naps. We laugh a lot.

I hope you won't find this chapter a doom-and-gloom downer. You shouldn't. Instead, learn from this smorgasbord of stories, and use it as a source of provocative solutions that can help you prevent your health problems from snuffing out your love life.

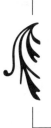

> *Old age ain't no place for sissies.*
> —Bette Davis
> (after suffering a stroke, double mastectomy,
> and broken shoulder over thirteen months)

Jane's Story

After decades of sexual abstinence, Jane, seventy-five, has fallen in love with Pete, eighty-eight. She discusses the joys and challenges of love and lust in later life:

> *I am a seventy-five-year-old female. I've been single all my life, and until recently, I had had no sex since 1968. I am now sexually involved with a widower, age eighty-eight. Our sexual need for each other today is as strong as if we were fourteen, but fulfilling it requires injections for him and estrogen for me for extreme dryness and narrowing of the*

vagina over the years. I never expected to make love again after an almost-forty-year drought (what a perfect word in this case).

After one month of trying, I am still unable to receive his penis vaginally—it's too much of a stretch, and, despite using estrogen and K-Y lubricant, dryness, yeast, and bacterial infections have plagued me. This is frustrating for both of us.

We have had oral and digital sex so far. It's both enjoyable and frustrating; I don't feel "together" with Pete without an orgasm of some kind, and I suspect only with his penis inside me will I feel complete oneness. I do feel togetherness when I can bring him to orgasm orally.

We absolutely feel sexy together. I'll take anything I can get from this man. I love him in every way. The most frustrating thing is my vaginal dryness. We're working on getting me a real orgasm orally, but he's having to learn my needs from scratch, and it's not easy to remember the perfect words to describe how he needs to refine his technique. Of course, he has trouble slowing down and lightening up enough. But he's an eager student. One of us worked in counseling, the other in medicine—a combination that makes for loving, knowledgeable coupling!

We live in a community of quite aged seniors who seem generally conservative and asexual. The number of subjects that must never be mentioned versus the subjects that are acceptable in conversation unnerved me enough to send me ransacking the community for the very few who spoke or at least understood my language. It's hard to find a support system about these issues.

Touching, talking, and laughing are important to us both, although he hasn't yet learned to appreciate the simple joy of touching. Outside of the bedroom, I want to touch him all the time we're together. I'm forever reaching for his hand or touching his white hair. He is much more interested in fondling me sexually, and while I'm responsive to that, often I would prefer simple tenderness, especially when I'm in pain. We both have serious health problems: heart disease, arteriosclerosis, significant memory loss, disk disintegration and herniation, pain, energy depletion, and more.

My sex drive is unleashed when we're both rested and know we can have unhurried time together. We have leaned the absolute necessity of being rested. Pete usually naps, and I clear my day; then we have late-afternoon lovemaking, another rest, wine, and a late dinner. My physical desire, when we finally have our clothes off and reach for each other, is overwhelming. At other times, whether we're together or apart, it's the bonding that counts most to me.

As for what women need to know about sex after seventy or eighty, that's simple: as long as the body's main sex organ—the brain—is operating, sex is always what you can make of it. A healthy person of any age can be as sexy as she or he wants. Pete's and my sex life is limited not by age but by chronic fatigue and pain.

I have many years of experience as a counselor, so I am better able than most to bring up touchy subjects and allow both of us to speak honestly and listen carefully. This

Sexually Seasoned Women Speak about Their Own Physical Challenges

Increasing osteoarthritis causes me to be less flexible. I have difficulty spreading my legs and need to find different positions for intercourse. *(Phoebe, 64)*

When we started, I saw my lover look off in the distance while we were screwing. I asked if I felt loose to him—I had had four children. So, I had surgeries to tighten my vagina, my bladder, and in between. That made a difference for him. *(Bea, 77)*

Last fall, I was diagnosed with bladder cancer. They removed a tumor. I freaked out at first, but then I learned about it and went through treatment. At my last exam, they couldn't find any cancer cells. I have to keep going back, and I hope they won't find anything again. That was an incentive to live my life. *(Claire, 66)*

is especially valuable because Pete is a late learner about women in general. I believe this stunting of emotional growth is extremely common in his generation. The brain may be the primary sex organ, but it can also be its own worst enemy. Geezers who fought their way across Europe and the Pacific sixty years ago still can't have good sex unless they can talk about it comfortably, eye-to-eye, with their partners—and too many have never tossed out the taboos they learned from their Victorian parents.

Bob's Story

You met Leona, seventy-seven, and Bob, seventy-six, in Chapter 13, "Late Bloomers—Ready to Fly." What we didn't share earlier is that Bob had heart surgery a few years ago, and since then has been taking cardiac medicines. "That was the end of erections," says Bob. "It didn't affect the libido nor the orgasm at all, but it sure as hell affected erections to the point where I can't get one unless I inject myself with medication. Because of the type of medications I take, I can't take Viagra."

Bob asserts that there is no change in sexual enjoyment, and his lack of erections doesn't stop him from having an intensely active, loving sex life with Leona and his other partners. Leona and Bob have sex about twice a week, and Leona says she is "completely satisfied" with the "hands and mouth" sex they have. It's just that intercourse is rarely part of it.

"My libido is certainly less in frequency compared to the past, but the pleasure is no different," says Bob. "I was surprised I could have orgasms without erections. I thought they went hand in hand. I've had prostate surgery, and there's some emission, about a tenth of what it used to be. But I can tell I ejaculate, there's no question. It was a revelation that erection, libido, and ejaculations are all separate."

Injecting himself to get an erection is "no fun," Bob says, "and if I happen to inject in the wrong place, it's a miserable hour or two of pain." So he generally doesn't bother. "If I can't have intercourse, that doesn't mean I can't have sexual union. Sex doesn't have much to do with the penis. It's between the ears, at the end of the tongue, in the finger, in the cuddling. Inserting my penis in a vagina is not the epitome of life. I'd rather use my tongue, quite frankly."

Sexually Seasoned Women Cope with Their Partners' Physical Challenges

Viagra is wonderful! People make jokes about it, but it produces terrific erections and gives men an erotic thrill. *(Joanna, 61)*

My partner had prostate surgery and doesn't get erections without injections. This takes the spontaneity out of intercourse. We do kid around and hug a lot, and he holds me when I use my vibrator. Our relationship is much more based on caring, companionship, affection, and stability than wild and pleasurable sexual abandon, like in my past. *(Phoebe, 64)*

I've had wonderful sexual experiences with men who thought, *Why bother?* because they couldn't have erections. Who cares if he can't get hard, as long as he's good with his hands and his tongue? The biggest obstacle is the man's insecurity: He thinks he's useless if he can't have an erection. The whole world is focused on that. The main thing is getting to a point that you really don't care if he has an erection or not, and making sure you get as much sexual pleasure as you want. *(Nina, 67)*

My partner is seventy-nine and has not had a climax for several years. However, he has a penile implant and he enjoys having sex very much. I have trouble reaching a climax too now, especially since dropping my hormone replacement therapy. However, these shortcomings have an advantage in that our lovemaking sessions almost always last for an hour. He has to be aroused for the implant to work. We take turns doing fun things to each other, and our lovemaking sessions usually involve at least six different positions. One of our favorites is with me on the bed with my bottom at the edge, and he stands on the floor. You need a high bed for this! He cannot ejaculate, but he surely enjoys the trip, and so do I. *(Melanie, 64)*

I enjoy oral sex and help things along with my own fingers, touching him while also nibbling on his nipples, which seems to make him aroused and quite satisfied. This gets him at least partially erect. *(Ulla, 61)*

It was shortly after menopause that sex with my husband came to a halt. He wouldn't talk about it. Ten years later, after he died and before I started seeking male companionship, I found out I had genital herpes. I suppose he stopped having sex with me because he knew he had contracted herpes and didn't want to admit it or expose me. The sad irony is that he went without sex the last years of his life, and I found out several years after he died that I had an unfaithful husband! *(Marsha, 65)*

Prostate surgery has been a big challenge for my husband. Getting through all that, restructuring our sexuality, reassuring him that I'm okay with how it is now (he uses Viagra and a cock ring)—all that took time. But I love the emotional connection we have, and that's the most important thing. Whether he has an erection or not is not a big deal. We kiss, we fondle, we talk, we joke. Most of the time, we can have intercourse, and if we can't, so what? *(Tina, 61)*

Throwing in the Towel

I promised you an upbeat book, but I also promised you candor, and it wouldn't be honest to tell you that everyone who responded to my interview solicitation had a cheery, positive attitude about the cards life has dealt her. Specifically, not all the women I interviewed were as accepting of a partner's inability to have erections as the others I've quoted.

Dana, sixty, wrote that her husband of eleven years is impotent and sex has gone (over three husbands and forty years) from "special" to "manipulative" to "sport" to "power trip" back to "sport," and it is now "mundane and unimportant."

At one time in her life, Dana told me, "There was no one I wouldn't consider 'doing'—the more the merrier." She had sex on office floors and x-ray tables, in elevators, examining rooms, meat lockers, meeting rooms, executive offices, limos, law libraries, and others' marriage beds. "No one, no place, was off limits," she says. "What a rush of power."

Now, Dana and her husband do not have an active sex life, nor does she indulge in solo sex. "I have thrown in the towel," she says. "I don't care to go the Viagra route; it seems so silly. If you can't, well, you can't!"

Her lover does "absolutely nothing" that turns her on, and when I ask what she wishes he would do, the answer is "ditto." What else would she like to share with women over sixty? "Hang onto those memories."

I respect Dana's decision to give up on sex and her partner, but I hope that other women faced with a partner's inability to have the same sort of sex as before will consider other options.

*I wanted a perfect ending. Now I've learned . . .
that some poems don't rhyme and some stories
don't have a clear beginning, middle, and end.
Life is about not knowing, having to change,
taking the moment, and making the best of it
without knowing what's going to happen next.
Delicious ambiguity.*

—Gilda Radner

The Middle of the Story

I have described Robert throughout this book as a vigorous, passionate, sensitive lover. Absolutely true. At sixty-eight, he has been lucky enough to have never needed a little blue pill. His body responds the moment his mind is engaged—which happens with a kiss, a touch, a special look, or a few days of separation.

But we also have another truth: Robert has leukemia and lymphoma. We don't know how many more years we will have together. Of course, no couple knows that—but a cancer diagnosis makes it harder to pretend we have "forever."

Robert is an intensely loving, life-affirming, contemplative man who copes extraordinarily well with his cancer—physically, intellectually, emotionally, and spiritually. And yet, there are times—of course there are!—when he gets depressed about it, such as when fatigue crashes over him like a tsunami. He has to plan our intimate times together days in advance, making sure he gets enough rest first. He has difficulty sleeping at my house—I twitch,

---

When I'm in the Mood and My Partner Is Not
By Susan Campbell, PhD

When I'm in the mood and my partner is not, I have several choices. It's very important to recognize that I *do* have choices when this happens! I am not a victim.

Even before choosing a course of action, I think it's really important to check in with myself about how I'm feeling. Am I feeling disappointed, angry, frustrated? Am I feeling hurt? Am I imagining that I'm being rejected or that he is "not that into me"? I always like to know what my mind and body are telling me so I can stay with my feelings long enough to comfort or soothe myself before taking action. I also need to notice whether one of my old childhood fears is being triggered, like the fear of rejection or abandonment.

Then, once I am centered and know how I'm *really* feeling, I might do one or more of the following:

1. Tell him how I'm feeling.
2. Reassure him that I love him anyway.

---

or the cat jumps on the bed, or my leg bumps into his leg, and the deep, nourishing sleep he needs is broken and affects his entire next day. So now most of our dates are during the day, after he has rested and while he is feeling fresh and energetic.

Robert worries that I am dissatisfied because we're having sex less often than we used to. "It's not about how much sex we have," I tell him. "It's the bonding that's important, the connection." Yes, I love my orgasms, and I love his, but if (when?) we reach a time when we can't bring each other to that intensity anymore, we'll still love each other and find ways to stay strongly bonded.

3. Ask him if he'd be willing to pleasure me. (For many men, if I'm turned on, this will get him in the mood real fast!)

4. Ask him if he'd like me to massage him or pleasure him. (For others, this approach works better.)

5. Tell him I'd like to talk about how we're both feeling about the fact that one of us is in the mood and the other isn't. And ask if he'd like to do this.

6. Appreciate him for being honest with me about his feelings.

Bottom line: I always use a disappointing or frustrating situation to get to know myself and my partner better. There are many ways to deepen the intimacy between us, and going through an uncomfortable situation together—while openly communicating about our feelings—is a very good way to strengthen our bond.

Susan Campell (www.susancampbell.com) is the author of Getting Real, Truth in Dating *and* Saying What's Real.

Robert tells me I could cut loose from him now and not have to go through with him what lies ahead. "We'd still be friends," he tells me. How could he even imagine that I could walk away?

"We're in this together," I tell him. "The only thing I couldn't stand is if you distanced yourself and didn't let me share this with you." I *know* beyond any thread of doubt that Robert and I must be together for as long as life gives us.

I know this book is about sex, but sex—and the quality of sex—*is* intricately interwoven with everything else about love, life, and learning how to be in a relationship, especially with the perspective of age. And as much as we'd love to think we're invincible, these bodies of ours make us look head-on at our own mortality. I know that you, my reader, are nodding an affirmation of this statement, as you're butting up against your own or your partner's challenges.

Beyond Body Parts

Robert surprises me with a gift of sexy, silver earrings—multiple little hoops that dance and shimmer as I move. "Is there an occasion?" I ask him, posing for him wearing only the earrings.

"No," he says, then changes his answer. "Yes. I just got my social security check." We dissolve in laughter at the thought of a so-called senior citizen cashing his social security check and buying sexy earrings for his lover as his first purchase. Then our giggles turn to kisses, and we make love.

Yes, Robert and I are still able to have a joyful, immensely satisfying, and vigorous sex life. But I'm also aware of the parts of sex that are really important to me—to both of us—that don't depend on erections or energy. I love it when Robert wraps his body around me, spooning me, as many inches of skin touching as we can muster. I love it when we kiss, whether it's deeply or softly, urgently or sweetly, mouths seeking or lips barely open. When we walk, we hold hands. He watches me undress—every time, gazing at me as if it's the first time. Physical lovemaking takes all these forms and is sensual and fulfilling.

I love giving Robert a full-body massage. Often, this turns him on and becomes full-body lovemaking. Other times, he sighs with every stroke, and I listen to his sighs as my own meditation as I tenderly touch his back, his calves, his feet. Later, I cover his body with my own, and we hold each other in stillness, then we snuggle. I am at peace when I hear his sighs become quiet snores—a lullaby that often puts me to sleep, too. This is making love as much as the frolicking, raucous sex we celebrate at other times.

Can the Love Generation say we're still having great sex, despite bodies that confront us with brittle bones, aching joints, flaccid penises, or cancer cells? Yes, we can.

Maybe it's not always the screaming-orgasm kind of great sex. Great sex is what's happening between two souls, two minds, two hearts—not just two bodies. Great sex equals love plus humor, understanding, creativity, and life experience.

Life is what we make it—always has been, always will be.

—Grandma Moses

Appendix A:
When and How a Physician or Therapist Can Help

If you're not having the best sex of your life, an appointment with your doctor should be your first stop—particularly if it's because of a health problem that interferes with libido, comfort, performance, or enjoyment.

Only a third of women over sixty-five have ever discussed their sexual concerns with their doctors, although ninety-seven percent said they'd like to, according to a report published in the *Journal of the American Geriatrics Society* (January 2004). If women didn't ask about topics such as decreased sexual interest or unmet sexual needs, doctors seldom initiated these discussions, the study found, and even when women tried to bring up the topic, fifty percent reported that their "physician did not seem to understand or be concerned."

Fortunately, physicians and other health professionals are becoming much better informed about older women's sexuality. They have to be—the Boomers have arrived!

I've discussed my own sexual concerns with my nurse practitioner and my physician, both of whom impressed me with their knowledge and were happy to help me. I know other physicians who are committed to helping women understand and resolve their sexual challenges—and, in fact, have told me that they are eagerly looking forward to sharing this book with patients.

If your sexual pleasure or responsiveness troubles you, real-ize that most challenges can be treated, so it's important to com-municate candidly with your doctor. Please don't hide anything out of embarrassment. Your doctor isn't judging you, and he or she has experience helping women with whatever concerns you might have: vaginal discomfort, dryness, lack of libido, difficulty reaching orgasm, and so on.

Take action as soon as you notice a change—don't wait until it's a huge hurdle. If you've been putting it off, don't wait any longer. You deserve sexual pleasure at this time in your life.

Doc Tips

If you fear you might get cold feet and avoid the issue when you're face to face with your doctor, state that the problem is "sexual in nature" when you phone to make the appointment, the National Council on the Aging (www.ncoa.org) recom-mends. That's vague enough so that the staff doesn't know your business, but specific enough that you can't back out!

Here are some more tips from the National Council on the Aging:

1. Before your appointment, think about what you'd like to discuss. Start with the issues you're most concerned about. Write a list, and take it with you to the appointment.

2. Be clear and specific when describing your symptoms. Describe the symptoms that are most bothersome to you first.

3. If you think the doctor doesn't understand what you're saying, be persistent.

4. If you don't understand something, ask the doctor to explain until you do understand.

5. If the doctor prescribes a medication, ask questions. How

does it work? What are the side effects? How will I know if it's working? How long will I have to take it before I feel a change? Will this medicine interact with any other medicine I'm taking?

6. Take notes about the information the doctor is telling you so you can review it later. Ask if there is a convenient time to call the doctor if you have additional questions or concerns.[1]

Physicians, as well as patients, are frustrated by the short time span of an office visit. Have a clear agenda of what you want to discuss. Keep the agenda short and sweet so that there will be time to cover all your concerns. Be ready with a quick, straightforward summary and the specific details that will help your doctor address the problem.

Hearing Aide

"Medical studies indicate most people suffer a 68 percent hearing loss when naked," I read in a magazine ad from the United Health Foundation and the National Health Council. The photo shows a man sitting on the examining room table in a doctor's office, naked except for the one-size-fits-nobody drape covering his lap. Yes, visiting a doctor's office is stressful, and you're likely not to remember everything the doctor tells you if you're anxious.

A good strategy is to bring along your partner or a friend as well as a notepad and pen. If you don't feel relaxed enough to talk, listen, and write at the same time, your companion can take notes for you. An extra pair of ears comes in handy when you discuss what you learned later.

Internet Research Do's and Don'ts

Doing research on the Internet is admirable, but avoid antagonizing or overwhelming your doctor by wheeling in a wagon-load of research. Leave the heaping piles of printouts at home.

Instead, present your major findings and concerns concisely in your own words. Make a list of the sites you found useful, and have just a few, brief printouts with you as backup—clearly labeled and highlighted. Don't force these on your doctor; just use them for reference as you speak.

Information from a university site or an unbiased, reputable medical site is more likely to be credible than something you found in a chat room. Realize that much of the health information on the Internet is without merit, and the rest might or might not be useful for your particular situation. Listen and learn—don't insist on your opinion unless you've had as many years of medical school as your doctor. I'm not saying you should see your physician as Dr. God, just pay careful attention to his or her analysis of the information you found.

(If you'd like to learn how to find and evaluate medical information on the Internet, I've written a whole book on this topic: *The Complete Idiot's Guide to Online Medical Resources,* available at www.joanprice.com.)

Seeking a Sex Counselor/Therapist

Perhaps what is keeping you from having great sex is not a physical issue but an emotional one. A good therapist or sex counselor can help you work through sex and relationship problems as well as other issues that affect how you feel about yourself and how you relate to others.

How do you know if you could benefit from therapy? Tina B. Tessina, PhD, psychotherapist and author of *It Ends with You:*

Grow Up and Out of Dysfunction and *How to Be a Couple and Still Be Free* recommends seeing a therapist when one or more of these situations are preventing you from flourishing:

• You have problems that you can't solve by yourself or by talking to friends and family.

• You cannot control such behaviors as temper tantrums, alcohol or drug addiction, painful relationships, anxiety attacks, and depression.

• You have serious difficulties communicating in your relationships.

• You have sexual problems or sexual dysfunction that does not go away by itself.

• You have violent or abusive relationships.

• You have a general, pervasive unhappiness with your life.

• You and your partner have disagreements and struggles you can't resolve yourselves.

Find a counselor who is supportive and understanding and with whom you can be open, comfortable, and completely honest. "To see a counselor and withhold information is the equivalent of taking your car to a mechanic and giving him false information about what's wrong," says Tessina. "The counselor, like the mechanic, is liable to focus on fixing the wrong thing."[2]

Helping Your Man

If your partner has erectile dysfunction, don't chalk it up to "old age" or jump to buy Viagra over the Internet. The first step should be a physical exam and medical diagnosis. I know that men often resist seeing a doctor for anything short of a severed leg. The idea of admitting to his physician that he can't get it up might seem about as palatable as announcing it at his class reunion.

Do whatever it takes to get him to his doctor. He may be taking a medication that interferes with erections, such as a diuretic, blood-pressure medication, antidepressants, or cancer treatments. Does he know that smoking decreases blood to the penis? Or that excessive alcohol consumption can cause nerve damage and erectile dysfunction? Diabetes, testosterone deficiency, prostate cancer treatment, and diseases of the nervous system, such as multiple sclerosis or Parkinson's, may also cause ED. Cyclists sometimes report temporary erectile dysfunction from long (more than three hours at a time) bouts of bicycling.

Your partner's doctor can tell by examining him and testing hormone levels what the cause might be and what treatment is likely to get him back in the saddle again.

If your partner's ED has no physical cause, it might be due to an emotional issue, such as stress, performance anxiety, or an emotional trauma, such as past sexual abuse. In that case, encourage your partner to seek counseling. It's never too late to learn, to grow, and to overcome problems that seem insurmountable—especially with you, his loving partner, at his side.

Appendix B: Resources

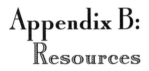

Books

What follows is just a sampling of helpful books on topics that concern women over sixty who are interested in having great sex. I've also included some excellent resources about sex for all ages.

We know that our feelings about sex depend a lot on how we feel about our lives overall. So, I've included some provocative books about aging, particularly women's experiences of aging, even when they don't deal much with sex.

I haven't included books that proclaim that particular hormones or supplements are the answer to health or exuberant sex after sixty because I don't believe that the answer is known yet.

I haven't included erotica, only because our tastes are all different, and an anthology that seems decidedly unsexy to me might bring you tingly sensations, and vice versa. There's plenty out there written by and for women, so you don't need to rely on my recommendations, anyway!

More books deserve inclusion, and new books are popping into our libraries and bookstores regularly, so let this list be just a beginning. What sex and/or aging books would you put on a recommended reading list for women over sixty? Email your recommendations (with comments about what you liked about them), and/or comments about my recommendations, to joan@joanprice.com.

Sex and Aging

Better Than Ever: Love and Sex at Midlife by Bernie Zilbergeld (Crown House Publishing, 2005). A guide to sexual enjoyment in the second half of life, including overcoming health challenges and staying sexy in long-term relationships, based on 145 interviews with men and women ages forty-five to eighty-seven.

Dr. Ruth's Sex after 50: Revving Up Your Romance, Passion & Excitement! by Dr. Ruth Westheimer (Quill Driver Books, 2005). Smart advice from Dr. Ruth about health issues, physical changes, and keeping your sex life with your partner interesting and fun, with stories of real couples.

The New Love and Sex after 60 by Robert N. Butler and Myrna I. Lewis (Ballantine Books, 2002). A geriatric physician and a psychotherapist discuss how physical aging, medical conditions, medications, emotional issues, and relationship changes affect sexuality. It's got a rather dry writing style, but it covers the ground.

Sex over 50 by Joel D. Block with Susan Crain Bakos (Parker Publishing, 1999). Frank self-help book aimed mostly at couples, with tips ("sizzlers") galore for recapturing romance and passion and plenty of anecdotes. Also deals with the sexual challenges of midlife and beyond.

Still Doing It: Men & Women over 60 Write about Their Sexuality edited by Joani Blank (Down There Press, 2000). Real people ages sixty-plus to eighty-plus bluntly and graphically detail what they do and what they like, including an array of sexual styles.

Still Sexy after All These Years? The 9 Unspoken Truths about Women's Desire beyond 50 by Leah Kliger and Deborah Nedelman (Perigee/Penguin, Spring 2006). Empowering self-help guide to understanding your changing sexual desire after fifty, with excerpts from interviews (www.womenbeyond50.com).

Sex, General

The Good Vibrations Guide to Sex: The Most Complete Sex Manual Ever Written by Cathy Winks and Anne Semans (Cleis Press, 3rd ed., 2002). Candid, upbeat, and friendly, this book is filled with tips for enhancing your sex life and descriptions of a variety of sex practices and toys. Explicit line drawings show male-female, male-male, female-female, and solo sex.

Guide to Getting It On! by Paul Joannides (Goofy Foot Press, 4th ed, 2004, www.goofyfootpress.com). At almost 800 pages, this hip, clever, and irreverent sex guide has everything you ever wanted to know and some things you didn't know existed. Graphic, witty, no-holds-barred.

Bodies and Self-Image

Fearless Women: Midlife Portraits by Nancy Alspaugh and Marilyn Kentz and photographer Mary Ann Halpin (Stewart, Tabori & Chang, 2005, www.fearless-aging.com/main.html). A wonderful book filled with beautiful photographs of fifty midlife women. See Chapter 4, "The Bodies We Live In," for a complete review.

Sex Toys

Good Vibrations: The New Complete Guide to Vibrators by Joani Blank with Ann Whidden (Down There Press, updated ed. 2000). Tips on buying, enjoying, and maintaining vibrators, this book is for both women and men.

The Many Joys of Sex Toys: The Ultimate How-To Handbook for Couples and Singles by Anne Semans (Broadway Books, 2004). A thorough and graphic guide to choosing and using all kinds of sex toys, not just vibrators. Also offers erotic stories and explicit illustrations.

Sex Toys 101: A Playfully Uninhibited Guide by Rachel Venning & Claire Cavanah (Fireside, 2003). A graphic guide to vibrators, dildos, anal toys, toys for boys, lubes, and bondage/domination/S&M.

Sexual Response and Satisfaction

Getting the Sex You Want: A Woman's Guide to Becoming Proud, Passionate, and Pleased in Bed by Sandra Leiblum and Judith Sachs (Crown, 2002). What's really going on in our post-menopausal bodies? Although there are only two chapters about women in midlife and highlife (as they refer to later years), these are informative and thought provoking.

Orgasms for Two: The Joy of Partnersex by Betty Dodson (Harmony, 2002). Discusses how women can achieve orgasms during sex with a partner, including the best positions and ways to include masturbation and toys in couples sex.

Reclaiming Desire: 4 Keys to Finding Your Lost Libido by Andrew Goldstein and Marianne Brandon, (Rodale, 2004). The cofounders of the Sexual Wellness Center in Annapolis, Maryland, lead you through an examination of your physical health, emotional resilience, intellectual fulfillment, and spiritual contentment, all of which affect libido.

Sex for One: The Joy of Selfloving by Betty Dodson (Three Rivers Press, 1996). Update of the 1974 classic why-and-how masturbation book, illustrated.

**About Men, to Help You Understand Him
or to Help Him Understand Himself**
All Night Long: How to Make Love to a Man over 50 by Barbara Keesling (Harper Collins, 2000). A sex therapist and former sex surrogate explains what a woman should understand about an aging man's sexuality, his "temperamental penis," and how to keep the focus on "lovemaking, not erections—partnership, not performance." Practical, frank, and helpful.

Great Sex: A Man's Guide to the Secret Principles of Total-Body Sex by Michael Castleman (Rodale, 2004). Castleman writes with warmth and honesty about issues that concern men at any age: their own and their partner's sexuality and pleasure. An excellent book for the man in your life.

Intimacy with Impotence: The Couple's Guide to Better Sex after Prostate Disease by Ralph & Barbara Alterowitz (Da Capo/Lifelong Books, 2004). A frank, practical guidebook to satisfying, sensual intimacy whether or not the male partner can have erections. An array of self-help strategies, from communication and creativity to medical therapies.

Making Love Again: Hope for Couples Facing Loss of Sexual Intimacy by Virginia and Keith Laken (Ant Hill Press, 2002). Candid personal narrative by Keith Laken, a prostate cancer survivor facing impotence, and his wife. Explores the couple's fears, arguments, resolutions, setbacks, and a new definition of intimacy.

For Men about Women, to Help Him Understand You

How to Give Her Absolute Pleasure: Totally Explicit Techniques Every Woman Wants Her Man to Know by Lou Paget (Broadway, 2000). Written by a woman, this is a man's guide to romancing, relaxing, kissing, touching, and teasing a woman for her sexual pleasure.

Satisfaction: The Art of the Female Orgasm by Kim Cattrall and Mark Levinson (Warner, 2002). Big picture book from *Sex and the City* star and her (now ex-) husband, illustrating ways men can satisfy women by giving them clitoral stimulation, mostly orally and digitally. (Not much to read, mainly look and do it.)

She Comes First: The Thinking Man's Guide to Pleasuring a Woman by Ian Kerner (Regan Books, 2004). "Cunnilingus should be every man's native tongue," writes the clinical sexologist in this straightforward, intimate, and exuberant guide to "the oral caress." Includes a multitude of positions and techniques, illustrated.

Aging and Women's Experiences

Age Ain't Nothing but a Number: Black Women Explore Midlife edited by Carleen Brice (Beacon Press, 2003). Forty black women writers, including Maya Angelou, Alice Walker, and Terry McMillan, write about their attitudes, bodies, and relationships in prose and poetry.

Getting Over Getting Older: An Intimate Journey by Letty Cottin Pogrebin (Little, Brown and Company, 1996). Well-written, provocative, introspective, often self-mocking reflections by the Ms. magazine founding editor, who tries to understand and "tame" the "gruesome ordeal" of getting older after turning fifty.

The Girls with the Grandmother Faces: A Celebration of Life's Potential for Those over 55 by Frances Weaver (Hyperion, 1996). A warm testimonial for "self-propelled," joyful aging. Weaver has written several books on this subject, all worth reading.

Juicy Tomatoes: Plain Truths, Dumb Lies, and Sisterly Advice about Life after 50 (New Harbinger Publications, 2000) and *The Juicy Tomatoes Guide to 50 and Beyond: Ripe Living, Passionate Women* (New Harbinger, 2006) by Susan Swartz. Warm and witty revelations and tips from saucy women who "revel in their ripeness" after fifty.

When I Am an Old Woman I Shall Wear Purple edited by Sandra Martz (Papier Mache, 4th ed., 2003). Aging women revealed poignantly in stunning photographs, poetry, and short stories.

Women and Aging: An Anthology by Women edited by Jo Alexander, Debi Berrow, Lisa Domitrovich, Margarita Donnelly, and Cheryl McLean (Calyx Books, 1986). Essays, photographs, short stories, art, and poetry depicting women's experiences of aging.

Sex and Women's Experiences (Nonfiction)

The Curse of the Singles Table: A True Story of 1001 Nights without Sex by Suzanne Schlosberg (Warner, 2004). Frustrated thirty-four-year-old writer recounts in laugh-out-loud detail her efforts to end her sexual dry spell. She's not old (by our standards), but we can identify with her mishaps.

Rescue Me, He's Wearing a Moose Hat: And 40 Other Dates after 50 by Sherry Halperin (Seal Press, 2005). Fifty-plus widow's adventures with online dating mismatches. Fabulously funny and often poignant. With dating catastrophes like these, single life doesn't look so bad.

Revolution in the Garden: Memoirs of the Gardenkeeper by Dell Williams and Lynn Vannucci (http://revolutioninthegarden.com/). Autobiography of the founder of Eve's Garden, New York–based women's sex shop, which the author wrote at age eighty-two. Her reminiscences include losing her virginity in a date rape in 1940 and attending Betty Dodson's masturbation workshop in 1970.

A Round-Heeled Woman: My Late-Life Adventures in Sex and Romance by Jane Juska (Villard, 2003). Sixty-six-year-old woman overcomes a restrictive sexual upbringing and places personal ad: "I would like to have a lot of sex with a man I like." She gets plenty of responses and trysts, but most of the results aren't very satisfying.

Sex and Sensibility: 28 True Romances from the Lives of Single Women edited by Genevieve Field (Washington Square Press, 2005). These well-written, frank, often funny narratives by women who are mostly in their twenties about their sexual experiences remind us of our own youthful escapades.

Still Sexy after All These Years? The 9 Unspoken Truths about Women's Desire beyond 50 by Leah Kliger and Deborah Nedelman (Perigee/Penguin, 2006).

Seeking and Finding Love after Midlife

Falling in Love Again: The Mature Woman's Guide to Finding Romantic Fulfillment by Monica Morris (Square One Publishers, 2004). An intelligent guide to dating after fifty, including where to look and how to enrich your own life, with many vignettes of men and women looking for love and a lively chapter about dating and matchmaking services. (Oddly, this book only has five pages about online dating.)

Older Couples: New Romances: Finding & Keeping Love in Later Life by Edith Ankersmit and Jerrold E. Kemp (Ten Speed Press, 2003). Fifteen couples who found each other in later life discuss how they met, how the relationships developed, and what problems they faced.

Seasons of the Heart: Men and Women Talk about Love, Sex, and Romance after 60 by Zenith Henkin Gross (New World Library, 2000). Dignified vignettes of women falling in love again in later life, interspersed with commentary and tips from the author about such topics as legal protection, emotional issues, how to relate to wary children.

Woman-Friendly Sex Shops

First, a definition: A woman-friendly sex shop is a neighborhood ("walk-in") or online store that celebrates women's sexuality by selling products that enhance women's pleasure: sex toys, books, videos, lubricants, and sometimes lingerie and racy costumes. The store or site is visually appealing to women, does not objectify women, and aims to make women feel comfortable there.

This means different things to different women, I realize. I have a thick hide, personally, but I picture a reader who has never visited a sex store before and try to imagine what her reaction might be. If she'd turn tail (so to speak) and run, it doesn't belong in this list.

To me, "woman-friendly" neighborhood stores have a friendly atmosphere, helpful salespeople who answer questions matter-of-factly but don't hover, encourage us to handle the sex toys (non-intimately, of course!), and treat sex as natural rather than sordid. They may offer seminars. The environment may be dignified or playful—never seedy. Personally, I am turned off by stores that seem to aim for young customers with loud music and a sharp edginess. That makes me uncomfortable, as if they're telling me, "You're too old to shop here."

I like websites that feel welcoming to women, offer an educational component (online guides or expert advisors, for example), and present straightforward information in either a dignified or a clever, friendly style. First impressions count: I am turned off by websites that seem to be leering or drooling and objectify women, with photos of body parts thrust at the viewer. I don't list those here, even if they carry the same products as the stores I do list.

I list stores that I have visited and sites that I have used personally. I also list neighborhood stores in cities that I have not personally visited, as long as they have an Internet presence that reassures me that they belong on this list. If you spot a store here that shouldn't be included (if it doesn't make women feel comfortable or it's out of business), or if a store you personally like is omitted, please email me at joan@joanprice.com with your comments, and we'll update the list in a future edition.

Note: All the following stores and sites specialize in sex toys and other sexual pleasure enhancements unless otherwise noted.

▮ CALIFORNIA

Good Vibrations

Three stores in San Francisco Bay Area and an online store: 603 Valencia Street (at 17th St.), San Francisco, CA 94110, (415) 522-5460; 1620 Polk St., San Francisco, CA 94109, (415) 345-0400; 2504 San Pablo Ave., Berkeley, CA 94702, (510) 841-8987 www.goodvibes.com (click Info Desk: Sexual Health/Product Info for helpful online articles)

The Love Boutique
Two stores, which offer products and home pleasure parties:
18637 Ventura Blvd., Tarzana, CA 91356, (818) 342-2400; 2924
Wilshire Blvd., Santa Monica, CA 90403, (310) 453-3459
www.loveboutique.biz

The Pleasure Chest
7733 Santa Monica Blvd., West Hollywood, CA 90046, (323)
650-1022
www.thepleasurechest.com

The Sensuality Shoppe
2371-A Gravenstein Hwy. S., Sebastopol, CA 95472,
(707) 829-3999
www.sensualityshoppe.com

Ultimate Elegance
Erotic clothing and fantasy wear
733 El Camino Real, Redwood City, CA 94063, (650) 369-6913
www.ultimateelegance.com

ILLINOIS

Early to Bed
5232 N. Sheridan, Chicago, IL 60640, (773) 271-1219
www.early2bed.com

The Pleasure Chest
3155 N. Broadway, Chicago, IL 60657, (773) 525-7151
www.thepleasurechest.com

■ MASSACHUSETTS
Grand Opening! Sexuality Boutique
308A Harvard St., Brookline, MA 02446, (617) 731-2626, (877) 731-2626
www.grandopening.com

■ MINNESOTA
Fantasy Gifts
Ten MN locations, see www.fantasygifts.com/stores/visitstores .htm for addresses
www.fantasygifts.com

■ NEW JERSEY
Fantasy Gifts
Three NJ locations
5101 Black Horse Pike, Turnersville, NJ 08012, (856) 228-7002; 731 W. Rt. 70, Marlton, NJ 08053, (856) 596-0676; 200-300 White Horse, Voorhees, NJ 08043, (856) 309-1008
www.fantasygifts.com

■ NEW YORK
Eve's Garden
119 W. 57th St. (between 6th and 7th Ave), 12th Floor, New York, NY 10019, (800) 848-3837
www.evesgarden.com

The Pleasure Chest
156 7th Avenue S., New York, NY 10014, (212) 242-2158
www.thepleasurechest.com

Babeland

Two NYC locations:

Lower East Side: 94 Rivington St., New York, NY 10002, (212) 375-1701; Soho: 43 Mercer St., New York, NY 10013, (212) 966-2120

www.babeland.com

■ TEXAS

Forbidden Fruit

512 Neches St., Austin, TX 78701, (512) 478-8358

www.forbiddenfruit.com

■ WASHINGTON

Babeland

707 E. Pike St., Seattle, WA 98122, (206) 328-2914, (800) 658-9119

www.babeland.com

■ WISCONSIN

A Woman's Touch Sexuality Resource Center

This site/store offers a wealth of women's sexuality information as well as products.

600 Williamson St., Madison, WI 53703, (608) 250-1928, (888) 621-8880; 200 N. Jefferson St., Ste. 101, Milwaukee, WI 53202, (888) 621-8880

www.a-womans-touch.com

▄▄ CANADA

Come as You Are

701 Queen St. W., Toronto, ON M6J 1E6, (416) 504-7934,
(877) 858-3160

www.comeasyouare.com

Good for Her

175 Harbord St., Toronto, ON M5S 1H3, (416) 588-0900,
(877) 588-0900

http://goodforher.com

Love Nest

Three BC locations:

119 E. 1st St., North Vancouver, BC V7L 1B2, (604) 987-1175;

102-4338 Main St., Whistler, BC V0N 1B4, (604) 932-6906

4687 Kingsway, Burnaby, BC, (604) 433-0112

www.lovenest.ca

Lovecraft

Two locations:

2200 Dundas St. E., Mississauga, ON, (905) 276-5772;

27 Yorkville Ave., Toronto, ON, (416) 923-7331

www.lovecraftsexshop.com

Venus Envy

Two locations:

1598 Barrington St., Halifax, NS, B3J 1Z6, (902) 422-0004, (877)
370-9288; 320 Lisgar St. (near Bank), Ottawa, ON, K2P 0E2,

(613) 789-4646, (877) 370-9288

www.venusenvy.ca

Womyns' Ware

Education as well as products.

Check out "Buyer Be-Womyns'Ware"—products the site owners feel aren't worth the money.

896 Commercial Dr., Vancouver, BC V5L 3Y5, (888) WYM-WARE, or (888) 996-9273

www.womynsware.com

LONDON

Sh! Women's Erotic Emporium

57, Hoxton Sq., London N1 6HD

www.sh-womenstore.com

INTERNET-ONLY SALES

Blowfish

Huge variety of sex toys and products. Read "Vibrator Buying Guide" for attributes of different vibrator styles, with photos of each product (www.blowfish.com/catalog/guides/vibrators.html).

(800) 325-2569

www.blowfish.com

Libida

www.libida.com

MyPleasure
Products and how-to and shopping articles about sex toys and other enhancement devices for women, men, and couples.
www.mypleasure.com

Red Ambrosia
Upscale boutique for "sensual accessories" for romance and seduction, not a sex-toy shop.
(800) 459-1897
www.redambrosia.com

The Xandria Collection
Expert Q&A as well as products.
(800) 242-2823
www.xandria.com

Appendix C:
Interview Questions for Better Than I Ever Expected: Straight Talk about Sex after Sixty

Do you wish I had asked you for your opinion? Following is the interview questionnaire that the women in this book answered.

If you're a woman over sixty and you'd like to be included in a follow-up book, please answer the questions and then send your answers back to me via email. You can go into detail when a question beckons, skip anything that doesn't relate to you, and add your own questions if you wish. Feel free to tell a story or describe a scenario that illustrates or clarifies an answer. (If you email me at joan@joanprice.com, I'll send you the questions in a Microsoft Word document for your convenience.)

If you are answering by email, please let your answers go on as long as you wish—pay no attention to the space between questions. Please use "Book Interview" and your code name as the subject header of your email, and send it to joan@joanprice.com.

Of course, you don't have to go public to enjoy and learn from this process of writing your own sexual memoir—you can fill out the questionnaire for your own private enjoyment and never share it with me or anyone.

Your identity will be kept confidential, and only your code name and age will be used to identify the excerpts used in the book. Please email me with any questions. Thank you in advance! Enjoy!

1. Code name—first name or pseudonym (for publication):

2. Age (for publication):

3. Real name, address, phone, email (for follow-up questions only, not for publication)

4. Would you call yourself heterosexual/lesbian/bisexual/other?

5. How active is your sex life?

6. Do you have a regular partner? If so, how long have you been together? Committed, exclusive relationship? Open relationship? Multiple/occasional partners?

7. What are the best things about sex at your age? How/why is it "better than you ever expected"?

8. What were you taught about sex when you were growing up?

9. How was sex as a younger woman different than now?

10. If you had a wild past sex life, tell a story from that time, or tell about a memorable partner:

11. After menopause, what physical/emotional/social changes challenged your sexuality?

12. How have you overcome these post-menopausal challenges? What did you try, and what finally worked?

13. If you had children, how did sex change for you when they left the nest?

14. Have you been single and in the dating game as an older woman? If so, how have you "looked for love" as an older woman? What methods/types of places/activities/resources/have or have not been useful to you? Please describe the challenges and frustrations as well as any joyful experiences. Feel free to tell a story!

15. If you're in the dating scene now, how do you experience attitudes of potential partners—how do they respond (or fail to respond) to your attractiveness and sexiness?

16. If you're not in a relationship right now, how do you express your sexuality?

17. Do you engage in solo sex? If so, do you find it satisfying? Feel free to describe what you do.

18. Do you use sex toys or other sex enhancers? If so, which ones? With or without a partner? If you've named your vibrator, what did you name it? Why?

19. How do you see your body now? What do you like best about your body, and how does this contribute to your feelings of sexiness? What don't you like?

20. Do you exercise or dance regularly? If so, how does this affect your sexuality and/or body image?

21. What challenges did you have to overcome to keep sex satisfying as you aged, and how did you overcome them? What ongoing challenges prevent sex from being satisfying?

22. How have your attitudes toward sex, your sexual activity, and your openness to experimentation changed over the decades?

23. At what stage were you the most sexually adventuresome? Tell a story from that time if you wish.

24. If you have frequented a sex shop, describe your experience. Please list any woman-friendly sex shops (walk-in or online) that you'd like to see mentioned in the book.

25. Describe something your lover does that really turns you on.

26. Describe something you wish your lover would do to turn you on.

27. Describe an erotic adventure you had after age sixty.

28. Describe a fantasy that turns you on now, whether or not you'd really like to experience it.

29. Describe some non-bedroom thing you do, with or without your lover, that makes you feel sexy.

30. How do you make sex enjoyable and satisfying if your lover is unable to have erections?

31. What do you do to spice up a long-term relationship?

32. What do you wish that women approaching your age understood about keeping sex stimulating and satisfying?

33. What would you hope to find in a book titled *Better Than I Ever Expected: Straight Talk about Sex after Sixty?*

34. What else do you want to share about sex after sixty?

35. What was it like for you to answer these questions?

36. Are you interested in submitting your erotic experiences, fantasies, or stories for a follow-up anthology? If you say yes, Joan Price will contact you later.

Legal release: I give Joan Price and Seal Press, an imprint of Avalon Publishing Group, permission to publish excerpts from this interview in *Better Than I Ever Expected: Straight Talk about Sex after Sixty,* in promotions for this book and in other articles, books, and speeches by Joan Price. I consent that my excerpts will be identified by code name and age only. Joan Price will keep my full identity and contact information strictly confidential. I give Joan Price permission to contact me for more information and to inform me about the book's publication and order discounts to which I am entitled.

Signed _____

Date _____

*(If answering by email, type "I agree" and your name.)

Notes

Chapter 1: Tale of a Book: How This Book Came to Be

1. Eda LeShan, *I Want More of Everything* (New York: Newmarket Press, 1994).

Chapter 2: Sex in the Golden Age

1. "Healthy Sexuality and Vital Aging: A Study by the National Council on the Aging," September 1998.

2. R. L. Winn and N. Newton, "Sexuality in Aging: A Study of 106 Cultures," *Archives of Sexual Behavior* 2, No. 4, 1982.

3. Sheryl A. Kingsberg, "The Impact of Aging on Sexual Function in Women and Their Partners," *Archives of Sexual Behavior* 31, No. 5, October 2002, 431–437.

4. Jonathan Margolis, *O: The Intimate History of the Orgasm* (New York: Grove Press, 2004).

Chapter 3: My Sex Education

1. Genevieve Field, *Sex and Sensibility: 28 True Romances from the Lives of Single Women* (New York: Washington Square Press, 2005).

Chapter 4: The Bodies We Live In

1. Susan Swartz, *Juicy Tomatoes: Plain Truths, Dumb Lies, and Sisterly Advice about Life after 50* (New Harbinger Publications, 2000).

2. Naomi Wolf, *The Beauty Myth: How Images of Beauty Are Used against Women* (William Morrow & Company, 1991).

3. Nancy Alspaugh, Marilyn Kentz, and photographer Mary Ann Halpin, *Fearless Women: Midlife Portraits* (New York: Stewart, Tabori & Chang, 2005).

Chapter 5: It Ain't Easy after Menopause

1. Kingsberg, October 2002, 431–437.

2. Joan Price, "Hot Flash Flashbacks," excerpted from "The Boomers Approach Menopause (Kicking and Screaming)," originally published in the *Pacific Sun* (Marin County, California), 1994.

3. Ellen Barnard and Molly Webb, "Painful Intercourse Problem-Solving," excerpted from www.awomanstouchonline.com.

Chapter 6: Fitness and Exercise:
Our Bodies, Ourselves, Our Sex Lives

1. Myrtle Wilhite, "Still Juicy: Maintaining Sexual Health through and beyond Menopause," excerpted from the column "Ask Dr. Myrtle," www.awomanstouchonline.com.

2. Cindy Meston, "Sex and Exercise," Quest for Advanced Condition, www.qfac.com/articles/sexercise.html.

3. Tina M. Penhollow and Michael Young, "Sexual Desirability and Sexual Performance: Does Exercise and Fitness Really Matter?" *Electronic Journal of Human Sexuality* 7, October 5, 2004, www.ejhs.org/volume7/fitness.html.

4. Katherine Esposito, Francesco Giugliano, Carmen Di Palo, Giovanni Giugliano, Raffaele Marfella, Francesco D'Andrea, Massimo D'Armiento, and Dario Giugliano, "Effect of Lifestyle Changes on Erectile Dysfunction in Obese Men: A Randomized

Controlled Trial," *Journal of the American Medical Association* 291, No. 24 (June 23/30, 2004), 2978–2983.

5. Read more about Kegels at www.a-womans-touch.com/article/0/42/Pelvic_Floor_Strength_Kegels.html.

Chapter 7: Public Sex Acts and Private Preparations

1. Leonard Shlain, *Sex, Time, and Power: How Women's Sexuality Shaped Human Evolution* (New York: Viking Penguin, 2003).

Chapter 8: Beds Afire: Stoking the Slower-Burning Flame

1. Sue Johanson, *Sex, Sex, and More Sex* (New York: Regan Books, 2004).

2. *Encarta Dictionary* (Redmond, WA: Microsoft, 2003).

Chapter 9: Plug In, Turn On: The Quick Version of Everything You Need to Know about Sex Toys

1. Carol Queen, "Your First Vibrator: The Possibilities of Pleasure," www.goodvibes.com.

2. Ellen Barnard, "Four Tips for Toys: A Guide for Women of a Certain Age," excerpted from www.a-womans-touch.com/article/9/118/How_to_choose_a_vibrator.html.

Chapter 10: Staying Sexy without a Partner

1. Alex Comfort, *The Joy of Sex: Fully Revised & Completely Updated for the 21st Century* (New York: Crown, 2002).

2. Myrtle Wilhite, "Vaginal Rejuvenation & Health," originally published online at: www.a-womans-touch.com/article/2/27/Vaginal_Rejuvenation_Health.html.

3. Murray A. Freedman, Department of Obstetrics and Gynecology, Medical College of Georgia, Augusta, Georgia. A full presentation can be found at: www.parentsurf.com/p/articles/mi_m0CYD/is_5_40/ai_n13472405.

Chapter 14: Sparking the Familiar Fire:
How to Spice Up a Long-Term Relationship

1. Dell Williams and Lynn Vannucci, *Revolution in the Garden: Memoirs of the Gardenkeeper* (Los Angeles: Silverback Books Inc., 2005).
2. Tina B. Tessina, *How to Be a Couple and Still Be Free* (Franklin Lakes, NJ: New Page Books, 2002), 231–233.

Appendix A: Doc Talk: When and How
a Physician or Therapist Can Help

1. Excerpted from "Seniors' Corner Health Tips," the National Council on the Aging, www.ncoa.org.
2. Tina B. Tessina, *It Ends with You: Grow Up and Out of Dysfunction* (Franklin Lakes, NJ: New Page Books, 2003), 124.

Acknowledgments

This book could not have happened without the enthusiasm and skill of my remarkable editor, Brooke Warner. Brooke is the ideal editor: immediately helpful when I ask for it and hands-off when I'm happy working on my own. She has been an absolute delight throughout this process.

I am indebted to the sexy, sassy women who gave of themselves so freely in their interviews. They opened up their private worlds and shared their thoughts, experiences, relationships, and fantasies with me—and, now, with you. I learned plenty from them, and so will you.

Thanks also to the experts who offered tips and to the wonderful folks at Seal Press who believed in this project.

I am grateful to the people in my personal life who helped me along my journey to this spot, especially Larry and Eda LeShan, who guided me and offered role models for living and loving deeply.

Above all, I thank you, Robert, for your love and support and for permitting me to share and celebrate our intimate life here. It is my great privilege to love you.

Credits

Excerpt from "The Impact of Aging on Sexual Function in Women and Their Partners," by Sheryl A. Kingsberg, PhD, originally published in *Archives of Sexual Behavior* (2002), is reprinted by kind permission of Springer Science and Business Media in Berlin, Germany.

Excerpt from "The Boomers Approach Menopause (Kicking and Screaming)," originally published in the *Pacific Sun* (1994), is reprinted by permission of the author and copyright holder Joan Price.

Selections from *Ask Dr. Myrtle,* the online column found at www.awomans touchonline.com, are reproduced by permission of the author, Myrtle Wilhite, MD, MS, co-owner of A Woman's Touch Sexuality Resource Center in Madison, Wisconsin.

Excerpt from "Four Tips for Toys: A Guide for Women of a Certain Age," by Ellen Barnard, MSSW, is reprinted by permission of the author and Myrtle Wilhite, MD, MS, co-owner of A Woman's Touch Sexuality Resource Center in Madison, Wisconsin.

"When I'm in the Mood and My Partner Is Not," by Susan Campbell, PhD (www.susancampbell.com), was written for this book and is published by permission of the author.

Selections excerpted from "Seniors' Corner Health Tips" at the National Council on the Aging are reprinted by permission of the National Council on the Aging (www.ncoa.org).

"Get Together" by Chester W. Powers, Jr. © 1963 by Irving Music. All rights administered by Irving Music, Inc. / BMI. Used by permission. All rights reserved.

About the Author

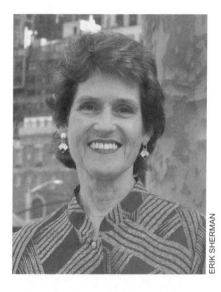

ERIK SHERMAN

Ageless sexuality advocate Joan Price is an author, speaker, dance instructor, and fitness professional. After one marriage, several serious relationships, and more flings than she wishes to count over decades of single life, Price found the love of her life at age fifty-seven. She wrote this book at age sixty-one to acknowledge the challenges and celebrate the delights of older-life sexuality. During the course of writing this book, Price and her fiancé, Robert Rice, decided to take the plunge and move in together. They live in Sebastopol, California, where Price teaches popular contemporary line dance classes.

For twenty-two years, Price taught high school English in Italy, New York, and California. Then, in 1979, after a near-fatal automobile accident, she realized that she owed her life to her exercise habit and had a mission to share with others the joy of movement. She left teaching, became an exercise professional, and wrote five books about fitness and health, including *The Anytime, Anywhere Exercise Book: 300+ Quick and Easy Exercises You Can Do Whenever You Want!* and hundreds of print and online articles. Visit her online at www.joanprice.com.

Selected Titles from Seal Press

For more than twenty-five years, Seal Press has published ground-breaking books. By women. For women. Visit our website at www.sealpress.com.

Above Us Only Sky: Essays by Marion Winik. $14.95, 1-58005-144-8. A witty and engaging book from NPR commentator Marion Winik, this collection delivers her trademark combination of searing honesty, unfailing wit, and down-to-earth wisdom.

Rescue Me, He's Wearing a Moose Hat: And 40 Other Dates After 50 by Sherry Halperin, $13.95, 1-58005-068-9. After losing her husband at age fifty-one, Halperin decides to get back into the dating game, with hilarious results.

Reckless: The Outrageous Lives of Nine Kick-Ass Women by Gloria Mattioni. $14.95, 1-58005-148-0. This inspiring book documents the lives of nine women who took unconventional paths to achieve extraordinary results.

Italy, A Love Story: Women Write about the Italian Experience edited by Camille Cusumano. $15.95, 1-58005-143-X. Twenty-eight women describe the country they love and why they fell under its spell.

Body Outlaws: Rewriting the Rules of Beauty and Body Image edited by Ophira Edut, foreword by Rebecca Walker. $15.95, 1-58005-108-1. Filled with honesty and humor, this groundbreaking anthology offers stories by women who have chosen to ignore, subvert, or redefine the dominant beauty standard in order to feel at home in their bodies.

Es Cuba: Life and Love on an Illegal Island by Lea Aschkenas. $15.95, 1-58005-179-0. This poignant and passionate travel memoir explores an American woman's love for Cuba and one of its compatriots.